Ayurvedic Zone Diet

THE ANCIENT WAY TO
HEALTH REJUVENATION
& WEIGHT CONTROL

Dr. Dennis Thompson
Edited by Susan Tinkle

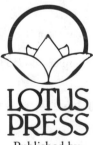

LOTUS PRESS

Published by:
Lotus Press
P.O. Box 325, Twin Lakes, WI 53181 USA

DISCLAIMER

This book is a reference work, not intended to diagnose, prescribe or treat. The information contained herein is in no way to be considered as a substitute for consultation with a licensed health care professional. It is designed to provide information on traditional uses of herbs and historical folklore remedies.

Cover Design: Irene Archer
Book Design & Layout: Irene Archer

For inquiries contact Lotus Press,
P.O. Box 325, Twin Lakes, WI 53181 USA
e-mail: lotuspress@lotuspress.com
web site: www.lotuspress.com
phone: (800) 824-6396

First Edition, 1999
Printed in the United States of America

Library of Congress Catalog Number: 99-75331
ISBN: 0-914955-85-3

Published by Lotus Press, P.O. Box 325, Twin Lakes, Wisconsin 53181

*This book is dedicated to the memory of my father –
we miss him sorely – to my mother who inspired me
through her dedication to her nursing career,
to my kids Cade, Shamanie, Fatima, and Shiloah,
and to my friend, Candice.
May God bless you all.*

TABLE OF CONTENTS

INTRODUCTION

Although it would appear obvious, for many of us the relationship and importance of health to other parts of our lives remain unclear. We know that to enjoy a life well lived, we must have our health. We miss so much when we are tired, or have a headache, or sleeplessness makes us sluggish. And when we are ill, we miss the opportunity to fully experience joy, prosperity, travel, a better job or promotion, even the love of our life – lost opportunity around every corner. Everything we do or fail to do is tainted by this comparison: what could we have done had we felt better, had more strength, stamina, energy? Health is the full battery that runs the toy, the giver of joy. It is the maker of potential, and the fuel that nurtures our greatness.

As with most things in life, once we lose our health, we value it even more. However, many of us resist taking the steps necessary to improve our lives. Of course, there are so many contradictory theories out there about diet, weight control, herbs vs. prescription medicines – so many 'paths' to good health – that we can become quite confused about just what to do and how to do it. In this universe, however, nothing exists without a cause, and good health is no exception. Therefore, a definable, understandable, practical approach to achieving a healthy body/mind (and keeping it) must exist. If only we knew what it was!

The Wholistic Principle of Ayurveda

In my experience, the best approach to overall, sustainable good health is through the application of the principles of *Ayurveda*. Though many wholistic therapies and practices exist, only two main philosophical paradigms are all-encompassing: the Chinese medical model and the Ayurvedic medical model. Though the Chinese medical model is excellent, I believe Ayurveda offers the best all-around practical approach to enjoying a healthy, vigorous life.

In this book, we will discuss the importance of wholism; the functioning of the body as a wholistic organism; Ayurveda's view of the body as *Vata, Pitta, or Kapha;* an overview of wholistic Ayurvedic practices for each body type; and the Ayurvedic principles relating to the body's ability to metabolize food. To arrive at an understanding of the way our bodies metabolize food, we must look at this concept of wholeness and delve a little into the way the body functions, its basics.

Body Types, Digestion, and Metabolism

From Barry Sears' recently popular book *The Zone*[1], I have derived the term "zone" when referring to the digestive capacities of the three Ayurvedic/Metabolic body types. Barry Sears' description of the zone is quite revealing; I knew the author was on to something that related to the body types described in Ayurveda. This book inspired me to look at the Vata, Pitta, and Kapha types in a new light. The zone described in Barry Sears' book seems to apply primarily to the Kapha body/genetic type. From my research, however, I concluded that *there is a Zone for everyone but not everyone is in the same Zone.*

The premise of *The Zone* is that everything in our life depends on what we can digest and what we can't. We can describe that capacity as our *zone of digestion*. Good wholesome food, if not digested, can and does create illness. We are not all blessed, however, with the same digestive system.

[1]Sears, Barry, Ph.D.; *The Zone: A Dietary Road Map*; HarperCollins Books, New York 1995

What works for one will not necessarily work for all. In this book I attempt to present a simple and practical way to improve our overall health based on an understanding of the process of digestion and how it relates to our body type.

According to modern medical research, the three basic body types known as *ectomorph, mesomorph, and endomorph* have different digestive abilities. According to the science of Ayurveda, the three basic body types known as Vata, Pitta, and Kapha also have different digestive abilities, remarkably similar to the model of ectomorph, mesomorph, and endomorph. These two paradigms converge with a study of the sympathetic and parasympathetic nervous system to produce three basic metabolic body types. This book will offer evidence that a particular body type can digest macronutrients (protein, carbohydrates, and fats) in ratios quite different from another body type. Further, there exists for each body type a "zone" in which health will improve or deteriorate depending on the ratio of protein to carbohydrates to fats consumed. When we know our own body type and its specific ratios, we can enter that area of optimal physical, mental, and emotional health known as the "Body Type Zone."

FOREWORD

The pursuit of the magic diet is an ongoing quest in the modern world. Indeed the role of food in health and disease can no longer be underestimated. The latest medical research clearly indicates the medicinal effects of food through vitamins, minerals and phytochemicals. Modern medicine is now waking up to the fact that natural healers have always known: we are what we eat. Food is the foundation of our physical reality and even our thoughts and emotions are closely tied to it.

Recent years have shown a plethora of diet books of all kinds. These usually aim at weight reduction as if that was the only real dietary concern. Most of them promote the same diet for everyone as if all human beings were of one type only. The limitations of this position are obvious.

Clearly, human beings come in many different types and sizes, with different temperaments, proclivities and activities. How can all these various, and sometimes contradictory, needs be dealt with by a single dietary approach, however well thought out it may be? Such dietary fads may sell well but eventually go out of style, just like fashion. They fail the test of time, which is why so few of them remain in vogue for more than a few years.

Because of the limitations of these mass approaches many people now see the need for a diet that takes into consideration the different types of people and their individual constitutional variations. The question then is what system of body types do we use to afford each person the appropriate diet? A number of new dietary approaches have come into being giving diets by type, which are defined in different ways.

Unfortunately many of these typologies are either inaccurate or incomplete. For example, there is a recent attempt to type people dietarily according to their blood type. While the idea sounds good and has some data that can support it, it fails the most basic test of observation. Within the same blood type we can find individuals of all shapes, sizes and temperaments—tall and short, fat and thin, active or sedentary, passive or aggressive. Does this mean that their blood type is sufficient to prescribe an appropriate diet for them? It has a point but misses the core issue.

Such mechanical typologies are easy and look good but do they work? Can the blood type determine what exercise a person should follow? The dietary type should also reflect the exercise type or it is not really dealing with the full physical typology. Yet blood type does not do this. Such incomplete or inaccurate typologies do not solve the problem and also end up foisting dietary stereotypes on people that may not be the best for them in the long run.

In the modern health scene we are witnessing the revival of traditional forms of medicine and their spread worldwide. These systems have many ideas and insights about diet. Of them probably none is as diet-based or sophisticated as Ayurveda, the traditional medicine of India. Ayurveda prescribes the appropriate diet as the foundation for all other therapies.

More importantly Ayurveda provides what is probably the oldest and most experientially proven set of body types. Its different doshic types explain simply and clearly the different types of people, not only physically but also psychologically. Ayurveda provides a solid determination of individual dietary needs and digestive capacity as well as the necessary sex, age and seasonal adjustments required to fine tune these.

Ayurveda has a well thought out food therapy relative to

its different body types. This Ayurvedic dietary approach is not a simple matter of phytochemicals but reflects an integral understanding of the elements and the vital force (prana) within the food. It understands food not simply in the abstract but the practical factors of cooking, spicing, and food combination. Nor does its dietary approach stand in isolation. It is integrated with exercise, herbal and meditation therapies offering a complete life approach to optimal health that is streamlined according to individual needs.

Dr. Dennis Thompson is a neo-Ayurvedic physician using the insights of ancient Ayurveda according the health concerns and context of the current culture. He examines important issues of diet, health and holistic living not only from a traditional Ayurvedic perspective but also relative to changing health and living conditions today.

I have known Dr. Thompson for a number of years. He came to a special Ayurvedic training that we offered in Santa Fe, New Mexico in 1993 and had been a student for some time before that. His enthusiasm and innovative spirit are obvious to all who know him. He has continued through the years to study and practice Ayurveda, adding his own unique ideas and approaches to this ancient system.

Dr. Thompson takes the insights of the Zone diet of Dr. Barry Sears. The Zone diet contains many important dietary insights, but lacks the constitutional basis of the Ayurvedic approach. Like many diets it is mainly anti-Kapha, targeting the watery or phlegmatic type person, and so deals with only one of the three main body types. Because Kaphas tend to overweight, which is the main dietary problem people address today, most modern diets are aimed at it.

Thompson finds the Zone insights to be valuable and in harmony with Ayurveda and takes them a step further. He outlines three health zones relative to the doshas or biological humors of vata, pitta and kapha. He shows how we can maintain the right zone or proper balance for our individual doshic type. In this manner he puts the Ayurvedic diet, which often seems ancient, esoteric or foreign, in a modern context and in a language where it makes sense and can be easily applied.

The book contains much practical information and well thought out regimens to improve health and vitality. It is not addressed simply to the health care professional but also to the ordinary person who is seeking dietary guidance and looking for a way to take control of his or her own health. Dr. Thompson's prescriptions take into consideration food, exercise, emotions and life-style and constitute a complete life-therapy. On the other hand, most dietary approaches in taking only food into consideration lack the full approach necessary to bring us to true health and vitality.

The book is one of the best additions to the Ayurvedic dietary approach. In fact it is one of the best new books on dietary therapy to become recently available. It also puts Ayurveda in a new and dynamic language that gives it a special appeal. Everyone looking for the right diet would benefit by examining Ayurveda, and this book is a good place to start.

Dr. David Frawley

Author of Yoga and Ayurveda,
Ayurveda and the Mind and
co-author of Yoga of Herbs,
Ayurvedic Guide

Chapter 1

THE WHOLISTIC PRINCIPLE

In our early years as a civilization we understood wholeness; it was evident as part of our culture. We saw everything as interrelated, part of a whole. We built societies based on this principle; most traditional medicines in China, Greece, Tibet, India, and even in our Native cultures here in the United States are wholistic in nature. While most ancient and traditional medicines are of a wholistic nature, modern medicine has shown a great tendency to adopt the opposite view – specialization.

Western medical science recognizes thousands of diseases and spends much of its time and resources trying to classify the treatment of each. This approach is riddled with problems inherent in trying to understand complex situations by reducing everything to parts, rather than looking at the whole. If we see the world as multiple forces moving back and forth without purpose or design, and we do not understand how everything fits together, the world takes on the appearance of chaos. We lose hope. From this perspective we cannot see the forest for the trees.

While a wholeness view sees the universe as one unit with many interconnected manifestations, specialization views the universe as having many unconnected parts. When we view the body from the point of view of specialization, we begin to see the body as a machine rather than an incredibly complex integrated system.

The Mechanistic View

The mechanistic view holds that the world is made up of things external to each other, which exist independent of one another and hold different ground in space and time. Their interaction with each other does not change their essential nature. For a more thorough description, consult Fritjof Capra's book *The Turning Point*[2]. The machine is the perfect example of this concept. A machine consists of totally independent pieces of material that do not change in their interaction with each other (unless, of course, to wear out). Each part is made separate and stays separate. Each part is at the effect of some external force making it move.

Our body, on the other hand, is a living organism that lives and grows in relationship to its other parts. The body constantly monitors bone density, blood chemistry levels, hormone levels, etc. and will shift properties from one area to satisfy the needs of another. The body is a perfect example of wholeness. Its parts are not separate; they cannot exist apart from each other or the rest of the body.

For the most part, modern medical practice looks at the body as a bunch of organs, glands and tissues that just happen to be in the same package – with little or no relationship to each other. That's why surgery to remove tonsils, appendix, the uterus, and millions of gallbladders has increased at such an alarming rate. Modern medicine does not recognize that everything in the body has a purpose and is part of a whole. When something as important as an organ is removed, the body is no longer whole. We can limp along rather well but the negative effects will stay with us until the end.

For all the surgery in this country, do we, as a society, experience better overall health? Can a new surgical technique be the "magic bullet" we need to become and remain healthy? Can a new drug or vitamin/mineral supplement, specially formulated from the latest scientific research, make us "well?" How about an exercise machine, will that do it? Probably not, because these fail to provide the key to sustained optimal health. The key to attaining and sustaining a

[2]Capra, Fritjof; *The Turning Point*; Bantam Books 1988

healthy body/mind is the principle of wholeness – understanding that the body functions as a whole unit, each part interdependent on every other part.

Whole vs. Fragmented— Order vs. Chaos

We all have different desires, goals, characteristics, temperaments, loves, hates, and preferences that give us the notion that we are different, separate. We think our bodies are separate from each other, that building is separate from the one next door, my headache is separate from my weight problem. The truth is that we are much more alike than we are different, much more connected with one another and with our environment—with the basic rhythms of life—than we are separate. The truth relates to our perspective. If we view the world as fragmented, our scientific experiments will show we are correct. If we can see that all things are connected, we can see each fragment and how it relates to the whole—where each piece fits in the puzzle.

We can see fragmentation, or separateness, only in the context of wholeness. If we live in fragmentation, we will see it as wholeness, which by its definition it can never be. If we see the wholeness, we will perceive the fragment for what it is—*part* of the whole, and not the whole. If our approach to life is through separation/fragmentation, then the answers we get to life's questions will also be fragmentary. We will see chaos rather than exquisite order. On the other hand, if we can see life as an integrated whole, we will see differing points of view as just different perspectives within the whole.

Fragmentation has permeated our society right down to our basic thought processes. So how did we come so far afield? Probably, as we learned to divide our universe into smaller and smaller pieces, we simply forgot what we once knew, that we were dividing a whole. That which was once obvious became obscured by new ideas that seemed right, *were* right, from our limited perspective. We lost our awareness of how we fit into the scheme of things, how the universe operates, how natural law affects all things, including us.

Natural Law and the Nature of Truth

There are countless theories about how the universe works. The object of science is to give us some stable data that we can rely on – but does scientific research always give us Truth? Is it Truth, or is it just a theory? A theory is an insight into the workings of some part of life or the universe; it is not necessarily true knowledge. A theory is an observation from a certain perspective. It may be true from that perspective, but taken as a whole, untrue. If all accepted scientific theories gave us true knowledge, then we would still view the Newtonian theory as true today. However, it is not – and it wasn't completely true when it was believed to be so. What we believe now is probably not Truth either. Accepted knowledge is true one day and not the next; Truth is always true. The question is, just what is Truth?

David Bohm, noted physicist, in *Wholeness and the Implicate Order*[3] put it this way, "Instead of supposing that older theories are falsified at a certain point in time, we merely say that man is continually developing new forms of insight which are clear up to a point and then tend to become unclear . . . there is evidently no reason to suppose that there is or will be a final form of insight (corresponding to absolute truth) or even a steady series of approximations to this." Bohm goes on to say "When we look at the world through our theoretical insights, the factual knowledge that we obtain will evidently be shaped and formed by our theories." In other words, we will categorize the data that we take in according to our own perspective. We put the new knowledge to use to support the theories we already believe.

How do we look at the world? Bohm says " . . . what is needed is to learn afresh, to observe, and to discover for ourselves the meaning of wholeness . . . what we have to do with regard to the great wisdom from the whole of the past, both

---

[3]Bohm, David; *Wholeness and the Implicate Order*; Ark Paperbacks, London and New York, 1980

in the east and the west, is to assimilate it and to go on to new and original perception relevant to our present condition of life." He goes on to propose a new way to look at physics. He calls it the Implicate Order. In this view, everything is enfolded into everything else. The opposite view, the Explicate Order, which is now dominant in science, suggests that each thing lies outside any other thing in its own space, and is not related. The implications for health are very important. The Implicate Order, or the wholistic principle, can make it easier for us to understand why we are sick and what we need to do to get better. Once we are healthy, it can help us understand what we need to do to stay that way.

Illness and the Wholistic Principle

Wholeness is about the interconnection of things; of parts with other parts, even if those parts seem unrelated. Our body is a web of interconnections, the total of which equal the whole. Any one part of the body is connected to the rest of the body through various pathways: chemical, structural, hormonal, electromagnetic, and through the nervous system. When we affect one part of the body, we are affecting the whole; a ripple in one part spreads over every other part. That is why everything we do affects everything we *are*. We may not have all our connections working properly, but they are there. We may not function as a whole, but we are whole and can't get away from it. The phrase "I don't have it together" suggests an understanding that all our pieces may not be functioning in harmony.

One way to look at illness is as a lack of connection or communication between various parts of the whole. Because the body is a network of communication lines among all parts of us, if one part is malfunctioning, another might be the cause. A symptom does not necessarily relate to the cause, but may be the effect of something to which it is connected.

Don't Kill the Messenger

Symptoms are part of a built-in feedback mechanism that continually shows how our body is doing. If we have no symptoms, we're probably doing well. If we're in pain, something is not functioning as it should and we need to do something about it. If we ignore the symptom, we're ignoring our own body wisdom. If we treat the symptom without establishing the cause, chances are it will come back, stronger and stronger, until the cause is found and eliminated.

When we sit on a tack the pain we feel is not from a deficiency of Tylenol™. People take aspirin and other pain medication all the time because pain *hurts*. It is understandable that we want something to shut it off. However, when we consistently do this with medication, we are essentially killing the messenger. We can think of symptoms as the messenger of inner body wisdom. If we look at it from this view, pain is the message that something is not right somewhere. If something is not right and is causing symptoms, we need to find out what is going on – then we can decide what to do about it. We find out what is going on by tuning in to our symptoms, tracking down their source in the body, and taking responsibility for getting rid of them *and* their underlying cause. That is why we must be able to distinguish the message from the messenger.

Body Wisdom

We know by now that we must approach any health problem from the wholistic view. Remember, our body is one unit made up of smaller sub-units that are all connected. A problem in one unit can and does affect other units. This includes the connection between the mind and body. The body's condition affects the mind; the mind's condition affects the body.

From a wholistic view, if the cause of a particular problem is not found and eliminated the body will degenerate until the negative effects accumulate on deeper levels, eventually causing a constitutional weakness that results in severe health problems. These become the chronic degenerative diseases that plague our population. Cures for these chronic diseases will never be found in a pill or potion, because for every positive effect a drug may have on a symptom, dozens of other potentially negative side effects exist that may be far worse than the original symptom. Toxins created from a deranged metabolism caused by chronic ingestion of drugs can cause a further imbalance in our system's dynamic equilibrium. This creates further degeneration, illness, and loss of hope.

Why is it the pills we took that once helped us quite nicely have no effect now? Why do we need more of what we used to take? Why does the problem keep coming back? The only answer is because we have not handled the root cause. Even remedies that are more "natural," or come from a natural source, may take away the symptoms and leave the cause.

Let's look at an example:

Mary came into the office with a headache. After examination it was found that she had a vertebral segmental dysfunction of the cervical spine and muscle spasms in her neck. The vertebral bones in her neck were not moving as they should in relationship to the rest of her cervical spine, causing the corresponding symptoms of headache and neck pain. After using a technique to relieve the muscle spasm and adjusting the cervical spine, Mary's headache was relieved, the patient was happy – until the headache came back.

Mary came back for more visits and her headaches began to lessen in intensity and to disappear for longer periods. That made us both happy – but why did they continue at all? If we did not ask that question, we would never get to the true cause of her headaches.

Mary wanted to find the cause of her headaches, the bottom line. She was willing to look in three major areas for the source of her pain: chemical, structural, and electromagnetic stresses (see Chapter 2 for further discussion). In Mary's case chemical stress induced her headaches caused by an intolerance to certain foods. When we began to look at her diet as a possible source of the problem, it became evident that her body may be unable to handle chocolate. If she stopped eating chocolate, her headaches left for good! On the rare occasions when she splurged, the headaches returned. Through a viscero-somatic reflex, the chocolate irritated her digestive system sufficiently to cause an adaptive reaction in her cervical spine, resulting in muscle spasms, vertebral subluxations, and eventual headache. In other words, by causing a muscle spasm in her neck that subsequently caused the headache, her body/mind was letting her know that chocolate did not agree with her. This is *body wisdom*.

Mary could understand this when she began looking at the possibilities. Are *you* missing some important "connection" which may be affecting your health?

Chapter 2

THE PROCESS OF ILLNESS

The body's prime directive is survival. It does remarkably well, if we consider the things it has to deal with. Getting sick is actually quite difficult. It takes much chemical, structural, and emotional stress over a long time for the body to break down and show signs and symptoms of disease. I am not referring to the acute onset of a contagious disease such as typhoid fever, smallpox, or plague. I'm referring to the chronic degenerative illnesses that are so common in our society at present.

Stress

Most of us assume we live a healthy lifestyle, but we may discount all the stresses of modern living that affect our health, and *all negative effects are cumulative.* Dr. Hans Selye, a medical doctor in the 1950s, is responsible for the term "stress." He recognized it as a pressure that exerts itself on humans, which comes in many forms; "bad" stress as well as "good." Stress is anything that makes a demand on us to perform in some way, to expend energy. We can classify almost anything that happens to an individual as pressure or stress. Exercise, if done the right way, can be a "good" stress; if done in excess, it can become "bad" stress. A good stress can be almost anything that nurtures us but requires work, activity, or change to accomplish. Bad stress begins when the nurturing stops and the activity begins to diminish us. For example: relatives or friends come to visit for a couple of days. We get the house ready, cook for them, enjoy each other's company, and have a great time – good stress. They decide they are having *such* a good time they will stay a week! Bad stress!

The body's way to deal with stress is what Dr. Selye called *adaptation*, or the shifting of stress from one system or part of the body to another. This is why symptoms seem to go away without any treatment and reappear later for no apparent reason. The more stress we put on the body, the more it has to shift to survive. Shifting stress spreads the stress out over a larger area so one area is not as badly affected. For example, if we are on thin ice, and we lie flat on the ice to distribute our weight over a greater area, we will be less likely to fall through. In this way, our system adapts, or shifts, stress to other areas to survive and function. If we injure a shoulder muscle and cannot contract it without pain, the muscles nearby will take up the slack as best they can. Since each muscle has its strongest contraction point at a certain angle, the "helping" muscle will have a different angle and therefore be less suited to the job. The muscle will eventually deteriorate from the increased workload. Constant adaptation and shifting of stress eventually weaken the system.

Three Kinds of Stress

The three basic kinds of stress that affect our lives on a daily basis are structural, chemical, and mental/emotional stress.

Structural stress is the musculo-skeletal adaptation of muscles and the skeletal system (spine). This stress adaptation results in muscle spasms, trigger points, and spinal misalignments that can cause neck pain, back pain, headache, shoulder pain, leg pain, decreased mobility, decreased activity level, and the general inability to do what we could do before. An auto accident, a fall, sports injury or any bodily injury, aging, or even mental/emotional or chemical stress can cause structural stress. Emotional stress can cause muscle spasms, and chemical stress can lead to aches and pains. When our body *adapts* to these aches, pains, and spasms, our structural system is weakened.

In other words, almost any stress can become a physical problem. Ignoring the pain caused by structural stress or masking it with pain killers can lead to degeneration of bone, cartilage, and muscle tissue.

Chemical stress includes food allergies, environmental allergies, nutritional deficiencies, poor diet, and/or a general toxic condition of the body. These may cause fatigue, headache, stuffy nose, digestive complaints, aches and pain all over, and a host of other vague yet significant symptoms. Poor digestion and enzyme deficiency are the primary cause of chemical stress.

Chemical stress usually causes fatigue and many vague symptoms that do not seem to make much diagnostic sense.

Mental and emotional stress may be our most significant roadblock to good health. Relationships with family (spouses, ex-spouses, children, siblings, parents), friends, and co-workers contribute to the quality of our emotional well-being. Co-dependency, dysfunctional family relationships, addictive behavior and other destructive tendencies create illness. Anger, fear, jealousy, sadness, grief, are emotions commonly experienced by all of us at some time. We feel an emotion in the body as pain, or restriction, or general dysfunction. Anger can cause us to tense up, causing muscle spasms and stress on the nervous system. Fear can cause gastrointestinal distress. Remember that everything has a cause

Wholistic Healing Rule #1:
Know How You Got Sick

It is important that we know how to become healthy, but knowing how we got sick may be even more so. There are several stages of disease that slowly, over time, wear down our resistance. *Time* is the operative word. It takes time to become sick. Usually only highly contagious diseases, such as viral illnesses, plague, or meningitis may occur overnight. Chronic degenerative disease sometimes fools us into thinking that we have suddenly become sick and can heal as quickly. That is not usually the case. Arthritis, cancer, and heart disease all take time to manifest. As our body gets sicker, it adapts to survive, robbing from Peter to pay Paul, and Peter never lets us forget it. Let's look at some ways we become ill.

How We Become Ill

Dr. Hans Selye, in his book *The Stress of Life*[4], describes three basic stages of stress which manifest into illness: alarm reaction, resistance, and exhaustion. The *alarm reaction* is important; it is what prompts us to run away from the tiger. The adrenal glands kick in, the sympathetic nervous system is engaged, and we are ready to rock and roll. We run away from the tiger or climb a tree, the danger goes away, we calm down and our body returns to normal. This is how it should be.

Nevertheless, if the stress continues, if that tiger is continually chasing us, our system has to engage more often, to a higher level, for longer periods, and we burn out. This is the *resistance* stage. To keep us going, our adrenal glands eat up many extra nutrients that they have to rob from other areas of the body. These other areas eventually begin to malfunction because they lack the essential components needed for survival. We continue until we can't continue any more. That leads to the next stage: *exhaustion*.

According to Selye, the exhaustion stage of illness occurs when the body finally runs out of steam. Nothing is

[4]Selye, Dr. Hans; *The Stress of Life*, McGraw-Hill, New York 1978

left to draw from. That which we need for good health has long been gone. All we have left is bone-tired fatigue. Does that sound like you or anyone you know?

Wholistic Healing Rule #2:
Know What Healthy Looks Like

What is Normal? What is Healthy?

If healing means restoration, we must be able to recognize when something is in need of restoration or cure. We tend to ignore our illness until it becomes a nightmare. To know when we are ill we have to know what it might look like and feel like to be healthy. A healthy body feels and functions differently than an unhealthy one. This sounds simplistic but it is true.

I ask my patients to complete forms that provide information about symptoms other than their chief complaint. For example, we may ask a patient to show whether he or she has headaches rarely, occasionally, or frequently. When a patient indicates occasional headaches, I ask them to tell me how often is "occasional." I have gotten some amazing answers. Many people who did not consider headaches their chief complaint answered "occasionally," but when questioned further told me they had three to four headaches *per week*. I have three to four headaches a *year*. That to me is occasional. If we think that three to four headaches per week is occasional, we also think it's *normal*. In our own family or circle of friends it may *be* normal – but it is not healthy. And, if we think that it's normal, we will have our headaches forever because we won't think we need to fix what isn't broken.

We take pain medication to get rid of headaches, giving no thought to the message the body is sending. Why is the headache there? Where did it come from? We need to ask these questions. Otherwise, we will always have headaches.

Remember, what is "normal" for you may not be healthy.

Wholistic Healing Rule #3
Put as Much Energy Into Healing
as Getting Sick

It is evident that we don't get sick very easily. It takes time and effort. To regain our health, there needs to be an equal force going in the opposite direction. We won't regain our health by eating brown rice, or simply taking a drug or an herb from the rain forest. We will need to put a concerted effort into getting healthy, at least as much as we put into getting sick.

The Process of Healing

"Healing" goes on in the body all the time as curing, regenerating, or restoring. Our bodies do the healing, not the doctor – though the doctor may play an important role. However, when we have overloaded our body with stress, improper diet, lack of exercise and all the other "habits" that lead to a breakdown in our ability to cure or restore ourselves, we need help. This usually requires a change in our lives. If we didn't need to change anything, we wouldn't have health problems in the first place.

Deciding what to change is the most difficult decision we have to make. If we have been on any health journey at all we will have heard of the need to balance ourselves and achieve "wholeness." Just how do we do that? Some teachers advocate one procedure, others a completely different procedure. How could they all work? Why do some things work well for another's problems but they won't work for ours? Everyone has an idea about what we should do. "Everyone" includes our medical doctor, who may know very little about nutrition, and our chiropractor, who may have more education in nutrition and natural health and know a lot about the spine and structural problems, but may not practice wholistic medicine. (Many chiropractors do practice "alternative" medicine, but it is not necessarily wholistic.)

"Everyone" also includes naturopaths, acupuncturists,

and nutritionists, all of whom may know a lot about vitamins, minerals, diet, meridians, herbs, etc. but do not have the license or the training to diagnose and treat illness according to most state laws. Also included are those who work in health food stores, friends in multilevel businesses marketing "nutrition" products, the uncle who dabbles in Radionics, the mechanic who swears by his mineral toddy, and everyone else who think they know the best way to stay healthy. Though all of them may have something important to offer – even life saving – they probably lack the philosophical framework necessary for the practical application of health principles for our particular body type and genetic makeup. In other words, what works for them won't necessarily work for us.

The Purpose of Therapy

By therapy we mean vitamins, minerals, herbs, enzymes, exercise, meditation, diet, chiropractic, acupuncture, drugs, surgery, massage, and so on. For most patients, the only real purpose of therapy is to reduce their symptoms. From the wholistic practitioner's point of view, the purpose of therapy is to reduce the imbalance and eliminate its cause.

All therapies and lifestyle choices affect the body to some degree. To determine if a particular therapy or lifestyle choice is good for us, we need to know what effect it has on the body and our particular metabolic type.

Two Categories of Therapy

The wholistic paradigm contains two main categories of therapy: Suppressive Therapy and Expressive Therapy.

Suppressive therapy is geared to symptoms only. The word "suppress" means to bring to an end forcibly as if by imposing a heavy weight – to crush, to extinguish, censor, or repress. Remember that the symptom is our body's way to tell us about the present state of our health. Listening to the symptom and understanding its meaning is vital to our survival. An effective suppressive therapy extinguishes the symptom. At first glance this seems to be the best way to go – we would all like to be rid of our aches and pains as quickly as possible. However, as we know, if we have not dealt with the cause of the symptom, the problem will return. This is why some people suffer from headaches every day for years.

When a fire is burning in the basement of our house, is the best action to open the windows to let out the smoke so it doesn't interfere with television? Would we put exhaust fans in the windows to suck out all the smoke? Would we just continue as though nothing were happening? No. We would try to find the *cause* of the smoke, then call the fire department to put out the fire. When we disregard or cover up our symptoms, we have a fire smoldering in our body's basement, and we are ignoring the potential for disaster. A suppressive therapy covers up the smoke but does nothing to put out the fire, which may eventually destroy our body through chronic degenerative disease.

Examples of Suppressive Therapy

1. Aspirin for headache, minor body aches and pains.
2 Muscle relaxants/pain killers for back pain.
3. Cortisone for arthritis, joint pain/swelling, etc.
4. Drugs for almost any disease (the side effects of drugs themselves can also cause problems).

Expressive therapy: To express is to communicate, convey, or display. This is what the body is trying to do through our symptoms. The symptom is an *expression* of an internal condition, a sign telling us what to do or where to go. Expressive therapy works because the body is successful in removing the underlying cause of a health problem. The body is the ultimate healer. All successful expressive therapies are designed to help the body heal itself by:

1. Removing internal and external toxins,
2. Stimulating the body's own neutralizing and cleansing processes, and
3. Nourishing the body's tissues with appropriate remedies for better health.

Wholistic Healing Rule #4:
Get What You Need

To heal, we need to have all the essential components for health. That of course is the rub. How do we know we are getting everything we need? How do we know we are not? What are we missing if we have a problem?

In 1895, there was a janitor in Davenport, Iowa named Harvey Lillard who had been deaf for several years. A healer in the town named D.D. Palmer examined him and noticed that part of his upper spine was sticking out more than he thought it should. He proceeded to push on the spine and it moved just a bit. Harvey Lillard felt a release, then suddenly was able to hear. *In 1895, D.D. Palmer adjusted the spine of Harvey Lillard and restored his hearing.* Chiropractics was born.

Of course, not all deafness is caused by pinched nerves and spinal misalignments. But Harvey Lillard's deafness was. Because he responded so well to treatment, we can suppose that spinal misalignment caused 95% of his hearing problem. For him, getting an adjustment was a magic bullet. It was exactly what he needed. However, for most of us there are few magic bullets. But then there is Mike.

Mike was a patient who came in with symptoms of impotence. We may not think he would end up in a Chiropractor's office for impotence, but in a wholistic practice any symptom is fair game. Mike was interested in Ayurvedic medicine and the help that might be there for him. I examined him carefully and recommended blood work and urine testing. Then, as is my routine, I adjusted him from head to toe and asked him to come again in two days when the lab results would be in. Before his next visit I went over his lab results and found nothing significant. This case was going to be tough.

Two days later, however, he came in all smiles. "How is it going?" I asked. "Great, everything is working fine," he said. After a few more questions as to exactly what was working fine, he assured me his problem was cured! I was surprised, although that kind of thing happens all the time in wholistic practices.

Many factors can be involved in impotency. Mike may also have those associated factors, but they obviously are not that significant. For Mike, 95% of his impotence was spinal-related. For him, the adjustment was a magic bullet. It was just what he needed. For others, spinal misalignments may be only 10% of the problem or may not be any part of the problem. For these individuals, another essential need may have to be found and met.

The point is, another person's needs are probably quite different from yours. What causes one person's health problem may be totally different from the cause of another's, even if the symptoms are the same. That is why your neighbor's headache may improve with chiropractic treatment and your headache does not. *Your* headache may be caused by food allergies, environmental allergies, or even inflammation of a tissue or organ causing subsequent muscle spasms and pain. Several causal factors are involved in most illnesses. We have to consider them all. That is why having a wholistic point of view when looking at our health is helpful.

All the things we need are all the things we need. We just can't get by with anything less and still be healthy. That is the whole picture and the understanding of the wholistic philosophy. We will never heal ourselves unless we give ourselves what we need.

Full Circle Healing

Not all of us have the same needs. Of the many vital components of life, some of us will need more love and nurturing while others need fresh air and clean water. When we begin to recognize our needs, we then must look at the therapies available to us and select the one or ones most suitable for our healing. Now let's draw some circles to illustrate this notion of "Full Circle Healing."

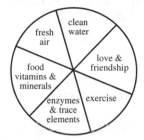

These are just some things we all need. We don't need them all in the same proportion, however.

Some of us need more love and friendship than we do exercise or even the basics of air, water and food.

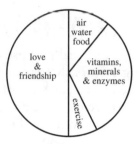

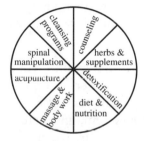

Here we have represented a few of the many available wholistic therapies.

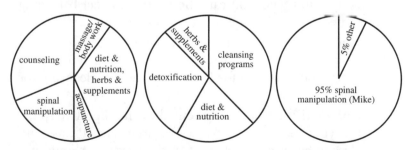

Of the many different types of therapies, one or more is just right for us.

Unfortunately, no omnipotent system exists to deliver wholistic health care by itself. Not medicine, chiropractic, or osteopathy. Ayurveda may be the philosophical paradigm that can give health professions a way to bring the various healing modalities together in a serviceable full-circle healing program for optimum health.

Wholistic Healing Rule #5:
Know What is Good for Your Body and Provide It

Macro (Larger) Perspective

The real purpose of any therapy is to treat the underlying factors that create disease. Once we understand that we need to balance our *dosha* (body type/constitution) on a daily basis, we come into the realm of prevention. Ayurveda is primarily prevention therapy, built on identifying our body type (genetic makeup) and following the program that nurtures our inner nature.

1. Take the tests in Chapter 13 to determine your body/mind type and see whether you suffer an imbalance of Vata, Pitta, or Kapha. You will also discover whether you need to detoxify your system, and determine if your digestion is too fast, slow, or irregular.

2. Choose balancing remedies. When you know your body/mind type, you can choose the correct balancing remedies and lifestyle practices for that type.

3. Choose appropriate detox remedies for your body/mind, i.e., colon cleansing for Vata types, liver and blood cleansing for Pitta types, lymph cleansing for Kapha types.

4. Choose tissue-nourishing remedies and digestive spices for your body/mind type. For example, Pittas who already have too much heat in their system should not consume significant amounts of cayenne pepper or

chilies. A Vata who takes a natural stimulant like ma haung or gurana may increase their already overactive metabolic rate. A diet of high carbohydrates and low fats might aggravate a Kapha due to increased insulin secretion.

5. Follow the appropriate diet, routine, exercise, body work therapy, lifestyle, stress management, and detoxification suggestions found in the complete Body Type Zone Program based on your body type. (See Chapter 14)

6. Commit to it. Tell others about it.

Chapter 3

AYURVEDA AND THE WHOLISTIC PRINCIPLE

Perhaps we need a "new" way to look at our health and disease. In India, more than 6,000 years ago, they formed the philosophy of Ayurveda for treatment of the whole body/mind. Ayurveda is the oldest known organized medicine on the planet and is recognized by the World Health Organization. Though Ayurveda has obviously withstood the test of time, we are currently experiencing a renewed interest in this philosophy of wholeness and sustained health.

The Basic Principles of Ayurveda

The Four Goals in Life

Ancient Ayurvedic wisdom holds that there are four basic goals in life. The first is *kama* or enjoyment. The desire for and enjoyment of life, of good food, of beautiful surroundings, is healthy. The desire to enjoy life is built into our system. It is a basic need. Desire sustains us. We eat because we are hungry. We enjoy beautiful things because they nurture us, and that makes us feel good.

The second goal of life is *artha* or prosperity. We need certain things to live, such as food, clothes, shelter . . . and cable television. This goal refers to our level of surviving in the world. We can't all go to the mountains and meditate;

some of us have to stay here and pump gas. Some of us only survive, and some of us thrive.

The third goal is *dharma* or career. For some of us this is the most important aspect of our lives. Doing the job we were meant to do is much more fulfilling than doing the job we have to do. Finding ones' purpose or career is so important it is life sustaining. If we don't find it, misery may follow us to work each day and back home again.

The final goal is *moksha* or liberation. This is the freedom to fulfill our potential, to express our inner nature to its highest level, to live life well. We can reach for these goals only when the spirit and body are willing. We need our health to have a life well lived. Good health gives us the freedom to be who we are – and that is life's true potential. That's everything!

Ayurveda and Universal Law

Over a vast amount of time the sages of India collected data about the workings of the universe. They concluded that all things have qualities, or attributes, representing states of matter and non-matter in our universe. They defined ten qualities and their opposites, for a total of twenty. We can describe everything in the universe from the point of view of these twenty qualities. Each is a characteristic or trait that affects living beings. These qualities, even today, affect every aspect of our lives. They are not stagnant, but represent a continuum from one possible extreme to another. Therefore, in Ayurveda, we can address health problems from the understanding of how living beings react to these qualities.

The 20 Attributes/Qualities as Essential Particles in Physics:

Heavy—Light	Smooth—Rough/irregular/sharp
Solid—Liquid	Slow—Fast
Cold—Hot	Clear—Sticky
Subtle—Gross	Stable—Mobile/moving
Oily/moist—Dry	Soft—Hard

Certain Qualities Fall Together

If we shake up a glass beaker full of water, sand, mud, gravel, and rock, it will settle out the same way every time. The heaviest (rock) will be on the bottom, the lightest material on the top. When we shake up the universe, the same thing happens. Things pretty much settle out in a predictable pattern, representing order from chaos. According to Ayurveda, these twenty qualities "settle out" in three distinct groupings:

Vata

Light, dry, irregular, mobile, rough, subtle, and cold qualities settle together in varying degrees. The Sanskrit word Vata, which means wind, was used to describe this grouping of qualities. A person with a Vata body type will exhibit more of these qualities. They will tend to be thin, with dry skin and hair, always moving about, complaining of cold hands and feet, may have irregular bowel habits, and may be a bit anxious about what is going to happen. If we routinely exhibit one or more of these qualities, we may lean toward a Vata body type, or be suffering from a Vata imbalance. The questionnaires in Chapter 13 will help determine your basic body type and any imbalances you may be suffering.

Pitta

For the most part, the qualities that represent the midpoint of the continuum were found to settle together as well: oily but not the oiliest, light but not the lightest, slower but not the slowest, faster but not the fastest. The Sanskrit word *Pitta*, meaning bile, was used to describe this grouping. Pittas will exhibit more qualities of heat and sharpness, but a more balanced tendency toward the other qualities. We could describe them as medium in build, medium in weight, intelligent, with a sharp wit, a good sense of humor, perhaps complaining of heartburn and tending toward irritability. If we routinely exhibit some or all of the above qualities we may lean toward a Pitta body type.

Kapha

The qualities of oily, heavy, stable, smooth, sticky, slow, and cold settle together in varying degrees. The Sanskrit word *Kapha*, meaning phlegm, was used to describe this grouping. A Kapha will tend to express the qualities of stability, heaviness, slowness, and dullness. We may describe them as heavyset, sometimes suffering from allergies and bronchitis, but calmer and more peaceful than the other types. They often have difficulty losing weight. So, if we are routinely overweight, if our skin leans toward the oily, if our personality/emotions are stable, we probably are a Kapha body type.

Vata	Pitta	Kapha
dry	moist	wet
light	heavier	heaviest
fast	slower	slowest
changeable	more stable	very stable
subtle	less subtle	gross
rough	smoother	smooth
moving	less movement	stagnant
jagged	sharp	dull
cold	hot	cold
hard	softer	soft

These groupings represent a way to bring order out of chaos. According to Ayurveda, we can classify all matter in the universe (including our bodies) according to the preponderance of these qualities in these groupings, with different percentages predominant. Try it. It may help you understand where you are out of balance and what is needed to get back in balance.

Body Types and the Five Elements

According to Ayurveda, everything is made up of the five elements, or five states of matter: ether, air, fire, water, and earth. Everything in the universe contains all five elements, but with different percentages predominant. Ether represents the source of all matter and predominates in things that lack density, as space. Air represents the gaseous state of matter; substances in the form of gas have predominantly air-like qualities. A Vata type has more ether and air-like qualities. Fire represents the power of transformation of matter; anything with heat or fire is predominantly the fire element. Pitta has more fire-like qualities. Water is the liquid state of matter; all liquid substances obviously have the water element predominating. Anything that is normally solid has the element of earth predominating, the solid state of matter. Kapha has more earth and water qualities.

The earth element gives the human body its structure and solid components. The water element is represented in our blood, lymph, and glandular secretions. The fire element is present in our digestive enzyme and metabolic transformation capacity. The air element provides our vital breath; ether, our spirit self. Ether and air combine to form Vata; fire and water combine to form Pitta; water and earth combine to form Kapha.

Ayurveda and Disease

Many similarities exist between Ayurveda and Chinese medicine. In Chinese medicine, the philosophy of polarized opposites (yin and yang) creates the paradigm with which to view the universe. A condition is diagnosed as either yin deficient or yang deficient. In Ayurveda, we diagnose a condition as too Vata, too Pitta, or too Kapha. Therefore, in Chinese medicine we might classify a person with heartburn as yin deficient; Ayurveda would look at this person as having increased Pitta, or fire.

Ayurveda's Six Stages of Illness

Ayurveda has a unique description of how the body becomes ill. According to Ayurveda the six stages of disease are: accumulation, aggravation, overflow, relocation, manifestation, and diversification.

Accumulation occurs when the local tissues start to become clogged with the residue of their own metabolism, in Ayurveda called *ama* (undigested food). The waste products of each cell need to be transported away for the cell's healthy function to continue. The wrong diet, seasonal changes, lifestyle changes, and other stresses contribute to this deranged metabolism. This stage of disease is the easiest to treat because it is local and not of great intensity.

Aggravation occurs when the local tissues become "backed up" with increased accumulation, begin to lose their own function, and start to apply pressure to the surrounding tissue. Organs begin to be stressed at this level but proper treatment can be very effective.

When a glass is full and we continue to pour into it, we see the next stage of disease, called *overflow*. This overflow now begins to seep into other non-related tissues, flowing into the blood, the lymph, and gastrointestinal tract. The disease is no longer localized; it is on the move, spreading to other parts of the body. This is a form of adaptation – the body spreads the stress around.

In the *relocation* stage, we clearly see symptoms. The accumulation of cellular waste becomes recognizable as a specific symptom, i.e., pain, headache, fatigue.

Manifestation is the next stage. At this point, we can see the complex set of symptoms as a whole and we can identify the symptoms as arthritis, asthma, diabetes or other specific diseases.

Diversification is the stage where the major element imbalance manifests its qualities. For instance, if Vata is imbalanced, the qualities of cold, pain, constipation, anxiety, etc. may manifest in the body. Symptoms of fever, inflammation, and irritation would suggest too much Pitta. Weight gain, swelling, lethargy, and respiratory problems would suggest too much Kapha. From these symptoms we can begin to decipher where our imbalances lie and how to correct them.

We can use these ancient Ayurvedic concepts to help determine what makes us sick, how to become well, and what we can do for ourselves to stay healthy. One of the most important gifts Ayurveda can offer is the understanding of body types. No more powerful information exists for bringing restored health to so many people. In Chapter 13 you will find questionnaires to help you determine your body type and define imbalances you may be experiencing in the here and now. Chapter 14 contains vital information as to your Body Type Zone Program – a regimen of diet, exercise, and lifestyle to bring you into your "Zone" of health and fitness.

Chapter 4

SOMATOTYPING: DESCRIPTIONS OF BODY TYPE AND PHYSIOLOGY FROM THREE VIEWS

For several thousand years, in many different cultures around the world, man has known that certain characteristics of personality seem to go with certain characteristics of the physique. Three basic approaches help delineate the differences in the basic body types. They are: Ayurveda (the study of Vata, Pitta, and Kapha body types); the study of the body as *ectomorph*, *mesomorph*, or *endomorph*; and the study of *sympathetic* and *parasympathetic*-dominant individuals. These three are vital additions to our understanding of ourselves. Somatotyping is the classification of bodies according to size, shape, etc., researched by psychologist Dr. William Sheldon.

In the previous chapter, we have begun a discussion of the Ayurvedic body types of Vata, Pitta and Kapha. Here we will look into Somatotyping and how it relates to these body types.

Ayurvedic Body Types: Physiology

Vata

The nervous system is the prime motivator of everything in the body. Its qualities are quick, energetic, and subtle transmission – Vata qualities as well. All muscle contraction is a result of nervous system transmission from the brain, down the spinal cord, to the muscle. When the brain sends a message to a muscle to move, it must get there quickly. The anterior and posterior muscles of the body must coordinate while we are walking and talking and going through life. When a muscle on one side of a joint contracts, another on the opposite must relax. This coordination requires spit-second timing, a Vata quality.

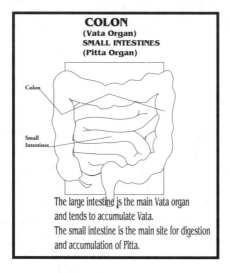

COLON
(Vata Organ)
SMALL INTESTINES
(Pitta Organ)

Colon

Small
Intestines

The large intestine is the main Vata organ
and tends to accumulate Vata.
The small intestine is the main site for digestion
and accumulation of Pitta.

Vata Organs:

1. The large intestine is the main Vata organ and tends to accumulate Vata.
2. The kidneys and bladder are Vata organs that eliminate the Kapha element of water.

3. The brain is a Vata organ whose main function is to provide communication between and organization of the parts of the body.

Pitta

The digestive system, which is the main system for changing substances into usable forms for the body, exhibits the transformational physiology of Pitta. The qualities of the digestive juices are hot, sharp, and liquid, which are Pitta qualities as well.

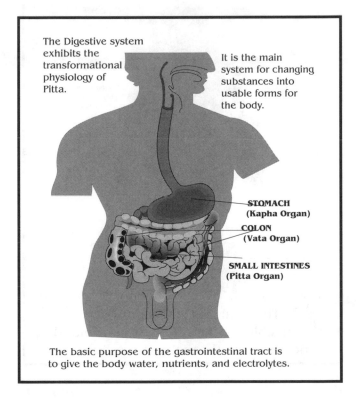

The Digestive system exhibits the transformational physiology of Pitta.

It is the main system for changing substances into usable forms for the body.

STOMACH
(Kapha Organ)

COLON
(Vata Organ)

SMALL INTESTINES
(Pitta Organ)

The basic purpose of the gastrointestinal tract is to give the body water, nutrients, and electrolytes.

Pitta Organs:

1. The small intestine is the main site for digestion, and the main area for accumulation of Pitta.

2. The heart is the Pitta organ responsible for the circula-

tion of blood through the system.

3. The liver and gall bladder are both involved in digestion and circulation. The liver produces bile that we store in the gall bladder until needed for digestion of fats.

4. The spleen is a Pitta organ involved in blood formation and destruction.

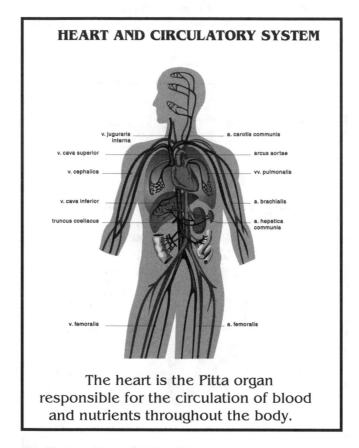

HEART AND CIRCULATORY SYSTEM

v. juguraris interna — a. carotis communis
v. cava superior — arcus aortae
v. cephalica — vv. pulmonalis
v. cava inferior — a. brachialis
truncus coeliacus — a. hepatica communis
v. femoralis — a. femoralis

The heart is the Pitta organ
responsible for the circulation of blood
and nutrients throughout the body.

Kapha

The body structure itself, including the muscles, fascia, ligaments, tendons, and skeleton, exhibits the stable qualities of Kapha. The qualities of the body proper are stability and cohesiveness: Kapha qualities.

Kapha Organs:

1. The stomach is responsible for digestion of protein and is the main area for accumulation of Kapha.

2. The lungs and respiratory system are Kapha organs responsible for getting oxygen into the body for cellular metabolism and elimination of waste (carbon dioxide).

3. The pancreas is a Kapha organ governing digestion of sugar as well as proteins and fats.

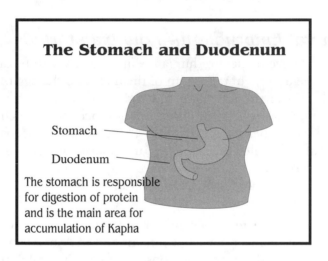

The Stomach and Duodenum

Stomach

Duodenum

The stomach is responsible for digestion of protein and is the main area for accumulation of Kapha

Cellular Activity

Vata, Pitta and Kapha also function within the cell. Vata manifests through the cells' connection to the nervous system and each cell's communication with other cells through the sympathetic and parasympathetic system. Pitta manifests through cellular metabolism and the formation of energy through internal cell structures such as the mitochondria. Kapha is the very substance of the cell itself.

Ectomorph, Mesomorph, and Endomorph: Physiology

Sheldon and Dupertuis studied the science of embryology and correlated both physiological and psychological traits based on the formation and preponderance of the three fundamental tissues that form in the body: the ectoderm, mesoderm, and endoderm. Using these tissue layers as a basis for constitutional typing, we can classify people as ectomorph, mesomorph, or endomorph.

General Embryology—how we started

The development of human beings begins with fertilization – the uniting of the sperm of the male and the egg of the female. From the fourth to the eighth week of embryonic development a process of differentiation occurs in which the cells divide repeatedly, eventually to become three separate layers of cells called the ectoderm, mesoderm, and endoderm. For purposes of this book we have only to know the tissues that are eventually formed and the functions of those tissues in body metabolism.

The *ectodermal* layer gives rise to the tissue structures that help us contact our environment and the outside world. These include the central nervous system, peripheral nervous system, sensory part of eye, ear, and nose; skin, hair, and nails, the pituitary gland, sweat glands, and tooth enamel.

The *mesodermal* layer gives rise to the supporting connective tissue structures which include the vascular system, the heart, the blood and lymph cells, arteries, veins, the urogenital system, kidneys, gonads, spleen and adrenal glands, as well as muscles, fascia, cartilage and bone.

The *endodermal* layer gives rise primarily to the gastrointestinal tract. During further development, the endoderm becomes part of the tonsils, thyroid, parathyroid, thymus, liver, pancreas, lining of the respiratory tract, and the lining of the tympanic cavity and eustachian tube of the ear.

These three different tissues are not equally distributed in everyone's body. Some people naturally seem to have more muscle mass than others. Others seem to have more sensitivity to their environment, while still others have more fat tissue and carry more weight. Thus, we can classify human beings according to the preponderance of one of the three fundamental layers of the embryo:

1. increased development of the ectoderm layer (which eventually becomes the nervous system) produces a body with more emphasis on nervous system activity, especially sympathetic stimulation, and catabolism (the breaking down of tissue), called the *ectomorph*.

2. increased development of the mesoderm layer (which eventually becomes the muscular and vascular tissues) produce a body with more emphasis on muscular activity, called the *mesomorph*.

3. increased development of the endoderm layer (which eventually becomes the lining of the gastrointestinal system) produces a body with more emphasis on the anabolic activity of digestion and assimilation – which leads to increased weight gain – called the *endomorph*.

Somatotyping

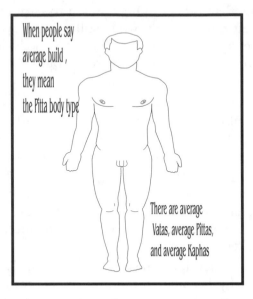

When people say average build, they mean the Pitta body type

There are average Vatas, average Pittas, and average Kaphas

Somato means body; somatotyping is simply assigning qualities to a particular body type: thin, medium, heavy, tall, short, quick, etc. Somatotyping can be further organized by looking at the embryological development of body tissues that results in three basic types: ectomorph, mesomorph, or endomorph. Dr. William Sheldon developed the descriptions of the ectomorph, mesomorph, and endomorph into a physical and mental/emotional classification system. A chiropractor named Dr. Robert Muller expanded on that work. In his book *Autonomics in Chiropractic*[5], Dr. Muller describes the basic body structure, chemistry, mental/emotional nature, and therapy considerations for each type. They are remarkably similar to the descriptions of the body types known in Ayurveda as Vata, Pitta, and Kapha.

The following are the basic descriptions of the ectomorph, mesomorph, endomorph, and Vata, Pitta, and Kapha body types and how they compare. Understanding each system will help us understand the other.

[5]Muller, Dr. Robert; *Autonomics in Chiropractic*

Characteristics of Ectomorph	Vata Characteristics
delicate build	underdeveloped build
spare, angular frame	thin, angular frame
stooped shoulders	prominent joints
narrow, flatter chest	narrow, flatter chest
long, lean legs	cold hands and feet
prominent joints	dry hair and skin
sharp, thin features	quick understanding
hyper-reactive to stimulants	but short memory
unpredictable	restless, active, spontaneous
sensitive to pain	imaginative and sensitive
poor sleep habits	poor sleep habits
chronic fatigue	frequent insomnia

Disease States of Ectomorph	Disease States Prevalent in Vata
tachycardia	nervous system disorders
hyperthyroidism	high blood pressure
gastralgia	anxiousness
arthritis & rheumatism	anxiety
neuritis	muscle spasms
cardiac arrhythmia	cramps
hypertension	insomnia
menstrual pain	poor digestion
Reynaud's disease	chronic pain
scleroderma	
diseases of the venous system	

Characteristics of Mesomorph	Pitta Characteristics
larger skeleton	average build
more muscles	medium frame
broad shoulders	muscular
wide chest	moderate weight
active in sports	good appetite
good coordination	aggressive
assertive	intelligent
energetic	sharp and critical
adventure-loving	courageous
Disease States of Mesomorph	**Disease States Prevalent in Pitta**
gastritis	digestive disorders
pancreatitis	ulcers
peptic ulcers	colitis
duodenal ulcers	gastritis
enteritis	heartburn
colitis	heart attacks
diarrhea	rashes
nausea	acne
inflammation	

Characteristics of Endomorph	Kapha Characteristics
large frame thick neck large hands rounded contours, round face tend to weight around abdomen relaxed posture slow emotional response calm, even temperament high stress tolerance need affection & approval	large frame gain weight easily carry more weight calm disposition peaceful receptive & open content, sentimental can become attached
Disease States of Endomorph	**Disease States Prevalent in Kapha**
mucous colitis eczema hay fever & allergies asthma edema arthritis most catarrhal conditions bronchitis cholelithiasis cardiospasm bardycardia hypothyroidism nephrosis migraine	chest colds allergies asthma diabetes obesity chronic sluggishness respiratory problems

Sympathetic and Parasympathetic Nervous System

We can also classify people according to the dominant state of *autonomic nervous system* balance.

The autonomic nervous system is made up of two opposing systems, the sympathetic nervous system and the parasympathetic nervous system. These two systems serve the body by automatically regulating and controlling its functions, and are generally not voluntary.

Let's look at the body as a hollow tube, the outer part being the skin, nervous system, and superficial structures, the inner part the basis of the digestive system organs. The outer layer is derived from the ectodermal layer of tissues. The inner layer is derived from the endodermal layer. Between these layers lies the middle layer, which makes up the muscles and connective tissue of the body. This layer is derived from the mesodermal tissue.

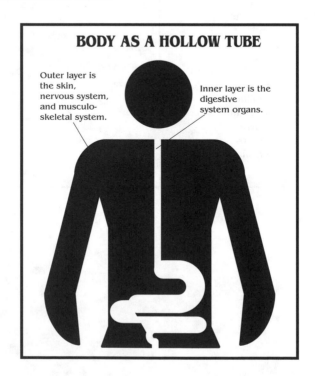

BODY AS A HOLLOW TUBE

Outer layer is the skin, nervous system, and musculo-skeletal system.

Inner layer is the digestive system organs.

The outer layer of the body (ectodermal) is activated by nerve impulses from the sympathetic nervous system. The inner layer (endodermal) is activated from the parasympathetic nervous system. The middle, or mesodermal, layer is activated by the somatic or voluntary part of the nervous system. While one layer is activated the other is simultaneously inhibited. When the ectodermal tissues are stimulated and actively functioning at a higher level, the endodermal tissues are more subdued. Conversely, when the endodermal tissues are stimulated, the ectodermal tissues are more subdued. Physiologically this delicate balance of activation and inhibition gives us *homeostasis*, or balance.

The function of the autonomic nervous system is to maintain the delicate balance between the organs of the body. It is when we disturb this delicate balance significantly with increased sympathetic or parasympathetic stimulation, that functional symptoms arise. Life is a constant search for a balance that is very fleeting. Once we reach this balance, it does not last long. There is a constant flow between activity and rest at all levels of the self. The body cannot continue in either mode forever. Rest must follow activity – systole then diastole. The heart beats, and it rests. Muscles contract, and muscles relax. We are awake, and we sleep. Our cells and metabolism swing from anabolism (the building up of tissue) to catabolism (the breaking down of tissue).

Mental, emotional, or physical tension usually speeds up the breakdown of tissue via the sympathetic nervous system. We register this tension in the soma, or muscles of the body. This indicates that the involuntary muscles of the visceral organs have been inhibited or relaxed and digestion is slowed. While we are eating or sleeping, our muscles relax and the involuntary visceral organ muscles are activated for digestion and elimination.

Under certain conditions such as stress, the fight or flight response of the nervous system can help define the physiological responses of each part of the nervous system. When confronted with stress, the sympathetic nervous sys-

tem becomes predominant while the parasympathetic nervous system becomes less so. If an individual is running away
from a tiger, survival dictates that certain physiological
responses are more appropriate than others. The body's
focus in sympathetic activity is moved away from digestion
toward the musculo-skeletal system. The adrenal medulla is
stimulated and adrenaline is released. The sympathetic division of the nervous system inhibits or reduces the function of
all the structures it supplies except the heart, thyroid, adrenals, the sphincter of the digestive and urinary tract (the
sphincter is contracted or closed). The heart rate increases,
the respiration rate increases, the metabolism increases,
digestion is discouraged, peristalsis is inhibited. For survival,
the body requires all its energy be focused on running away
from that tiger

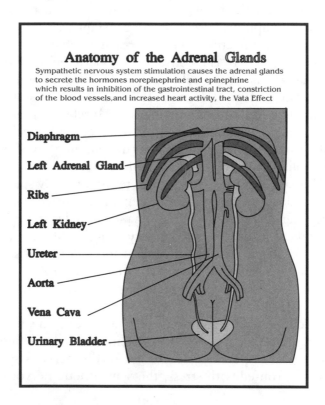

Anatomy of the Adrenal Glands

Sympathetic nervous system stimulation causes the adrenal glands
to secrete the hormones norepinephrine and epinephrine
which results in inhibition of the gastrointestinal tract, constriction
of the blood vessels,and increased heart activity, the Vata Effect

Diaphragm

Left Adrenal Gland

Ribs

Left Kidney

Ureter

Aorta

Vena Cava

Urinary Bladder

When the body is relaxed or in repose, the opposite occurs. When at rest, parasympathetic activity increases all the structures it supplies except the heart, thyroid, adrenals, and the sphincters of digestive and urinary tract, which are relaxed or dilated. The heart rate decreases, the basal metabolic rate decreases, the pupils contract, overall digestion and secretion of enzymes are encouraged, peristalsis is favored. The following is a list of the responses and functions of each type.

Sympathetic Nervous System Increase:
- dilation of pupils
- protrusion of the eyeball
- lessened gastrointestinal digestive enzymes
- lessened salivary secretions in the mouth
- lessened lacrimal secretions of eyes
- lessened mucous secretion of nose and throat
- irregular digestion
- lessened digestive tract motility
- . lessened peristalsis
- constipation
- contraction of sphincter
- increased adrenal secretion
- increased thyroid secretion
- increased overall metabolic rate
- slight nervous system tremor
- rapid pulse
- diminished urine output

Parasympathetic Nervous System Increase:
- contraction of pupils
- relaxed eyes
- increased secretion of digestive enzymes
- increased salivary secretions in the mouth

- increased lacrimal secretion of the eyes
- increased mucous secretion in the nose and throat
- slower but regular digestion
- slower but steady digestive tract motility
- increased peristalsis
- relaxing of sphincter
- decreased adrenal secretions
- decreased thyroid secretions
- decreased overall metabolic rates
- calmer nervous system
- lower pulse
- . increased bronchial secretions
- increased blood sugar

We would call a person with increased function of the sympathetic nervous system a sympathetic-dominant type. We would call a person who has increased function of the parasympathetic nervous system a parasympathetic-dominant type. The sympathetic-dominant type corresponds to the Vata and ectomorph body types. Co-activation of both sympathetic and parasympathetic systems corresponds to the Pitta and mesomorph body types. The parasympathetic-dominant type corresponds to the Kapha and endomorph body types.

- The Vata/ectomorph/sympathetic-dominant type tends to have more sympathetic activity of the nervous system (see listing above).
- The Pitta/mesomorph/sym-para type tends to have a co-activation of the sympathetic and parasympathetic system activity with possible emphasis on increased amplitude and power, resulting in a hotter and more powerful digestive system.
- The Kapha/endomorph/parasympathetic-dominant type tends to have more parasympathetic activity of the nervous system.

Summary of Descriptions of Body Type and Physiology

The three basic Ayurvedic body types are Vata, Pitta, and Kapha. These classifications are quite similar to the somatotyping that Sheldon called ectomorph, mesomorph, and endomorph. The common classification of bodies as sympathetic-dominant or parasympathetic-dominant also is remarkably similar. By combining the physiological descriptions of each system we can get a better picture of the whole:

Metabolic Type I: Vata type, Ectomorph, Sympathetic Dominant

Metabolic Type II: Pitta type, Mesomorph, Sym-Para Co-activation

Metabolic Type III: Kapha type, Endomorph, Parasympathetic Dominant

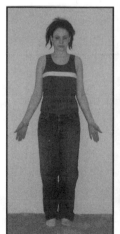 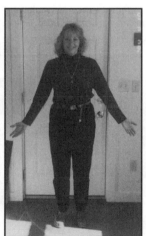 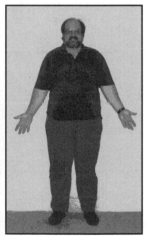

Vata	*Pitta*	*Kapha*

	Comparison of Major Characteristics of Metabolic Body Types		
	Metabolic Type I	**Metabolic Type II**	**Metabolic Type III**
Ayurveda	Vata	Pitta	Kapha
Embryological	Ectomorph	Mesomorph	Endomorph
Physiological	Catabolic	Transformational	Anabolic
Neurological	Sympathetic dominant	Sym/Para co-activation	Parasympathetic dominant
Chemical	Tissues Acid	Ionic Balance	Tissues Alkaline
Psychological	Enthusiastic	Fiery, aggressive, determined	Calm, peaceful, lethargic
General Physique	Lean/thin anxious/fearful	Muscular/ medium build	Stout/ heavier

Prevalent Disease States by Metabolic Type		
Metabolic Type I	**Metabolic Type II**	**Metabolic Type III**
tachycardia	_____	bradycardia
hyperthyroidism	_____	hypothyroidism
spastic colon	colitis	mucous colitis
gastraglia	heartburn/ulcers	_____
nervous system disorders	liver/gall bladder disorders	respiratory/pancreas disorders
hyperadrenia	_____	hypoadrenia
arthritis	inflammation	_____
hypertension	hypertension	hypotension
menstrual pain	cramps	menorrhagia
constipation	diarrhea	_____
insomnia	_____	_____
irregular digestion	_____	_____
anorexia	_____	obesity
problems with protein metabolism	problems with fat metabolism	problems with carbohydrate metabolism

Summary

Many cultures over the centuries have classified humans according to body physiology, or "type." Ayurveda gives us the basic body types of Vata, Pitta, and Kapha, which correlate with the more modern descriptions of ectomorph, mesomorph, and endomorph. As well, these can be correlated with the divisions of the autonomic nervous system (the sympathetic and parasympathetic).

The physiology of the Vata corresponds to the physiology of the ectomorph and the sympathetic-dominant type. The physiology of the Kapha corresponds to the physiology of the endomorph and parasympathetic type. The physiology of the Pitta corresponds to the physiology of the mesomorph and a co-activation of both the sympathetic and parasympathetic systems.

When we combine all three systems of classification and see their correspondences, we can better understand the ancient teachings of Ayurveda in the newer light of modern physiology.

Chapter 5

BIOLOGICAL CONTROL SYSTEMS AND THE ZONES

Physiology's main goal is to explain how the body works and the chemical and physical factors responsible for the development and continuance of life. Guyten's *Textbook of Medical Physiology*[6] states " . . . the very fact that we remain alive is almost beyond our own control, for hunger makes us seek food and fear makes us seek refuge. Sensations of cold make us provide warmth, and other forces cause us to seek fellowship and to reproduce. Thus the human being is actually an automaton." This is not to suggest that humans are machines, only that we operate in large part from automatic reflexes built into our system. These reflexes keep us alive without our having to think about them. However, most of our symptoms and disease processes eventually affect these mechanisms. That is why following a path recognized to be beneficial for our individual body type is so important.

How the Body Works

The body contains about 100 trillion cells. Though they all have different functions, they have certain similar characteristics. In all of them, oxygen combines with the products of protein, carbohydrate, and fat metabolism to release the energy necessary to run the cell and keep it alive.

[6]Guyton, Arthur C., M.D. and John E. Hall, Ph.D.; *Textbook of Medical Physiology*, Ninth Edition; W.B. Saunders Company, Philadelphia, Pennsylvania 1956-1996

Extracellular and Intracellular Fluid

We call the fluid outside the cell extracellular; inside the cells we call it intracellular. The goal of digestion is to break down the larger (macro) molecules of protein, carbohydrate, and fat so they can eventually penetrate the extracellular fluid surrounding the cell. From there, the cell exchanges what is inside (intracellular fluid) for what is outside (extracellular fluid). So the food we eat goes from big chunks to smaller pieces to the eventual microscopic size necessary to pass through the openings in our cell walls. The feeding of the cell is really the whole purpose of our entire digestive system.

The extracellular fluid contains nutrients for cell metabolism such as oxygen, amino acids, fatty acids and, of course, glucose. It also contains large amounts of the necessary sodium, chloride, and bicarbonate ions as well as the waste material of cellular metabolism, carbon dioxide. The intracellular fluid contains ions of potassium, magnesium, and phosphate. Several different transport mechanisms are involved in the exchange of these vital nutrients across the cell wall.

Homeostatic Mechanisms—Western Science/ Ayurveda

Homeostasis is the maintaining of constant conditions required for a healthy internal environment. Guyten states, "Essentially all of the organs and tissues of the body perform functions that help to maintain these constant conditions. For instance, the lungs provide oxygen to the extracellular fluid to replenish continually the oxygen that the cells are using, the kidneys maintain constant ion concentrations, and the gastrointestinal system provides nutrients." Homeostasis is the main functional operating system that keeps us all going. Without it, nothing works well – and eventually nothing works at all. Homeostasis is embodied in the wholistic philosophy that asserts that all things are interconnected.

Neural Control Mechanisms—Western Science/Ayurveda

The nervous system is composed of three parts: the central nervous system, the sensory/input division, and the motor/output division. The central nervous system is composed of the brain and the spinal cord. The sensory/input division is composed of sensory receptors in all parts of the body – the eyes, ears, nose, and skin receptors that constantly relay information back to the central nervous system for data processing and responses to stimuli. Appropriate signals are sent through the motor/output division to carry out the body's desires.

A large portion of the nervous system is under the control of the autonomic nervous system. The autonomic nervous system has two distinct divisions: the sympathetic and parasympathetic nervous systems (see Chapter 4). Essentially, the autonomic nervous system is responsible for all of the bodily functions over which we have no conscious control. It operates at the subconscious level and controls many internal organs, from the pumping of the heart to elimination of wastes. The body is "hooked up" to itself through this incredible system of nerves. Internal communication occurs through the nervous system. In Ayurveda, the Vata qualities of light, subtle, quick, and changeable primarily represent the nervous system. Symptoms affecting the nervous system may reflect a Vata imbalance.

Hormonal Control Mechanisms—Western Science/Ayurveda

Eight major endocrine glands in the body secrete chemicals called hormones. The nervous system primarily regulates the muscular and secretory activities of the body, while the hormonal system regulates metabolism. The hormones are carried in the extracellular fluid to the entire body to affect cellular function. The pancreas secretes insulin that controls carbohydrate metabolism. The thyroid gland secretes a thyroid hormone that increases the metabolic rate of all cells. The adrenal glands secrete an adrenocortical hormone that controls potassium, sodium, and protein metabolism. The parathyroid secretes a hormone that controls bone calcium levels.

In Ayurveda, the metabolism of carbohydrates is a Kapha Effect; the metabolic rate of cells is a Vata and Pitta Effect; protein metabolism, and control of potassium and sodium, is a Pitta Effect; and bone calcium levels are the Kapha Effect. I use the term "Vata Effect, Pitta Effect," etc. to describe those symptoms, conditions, qualities, and general tendencies attributed to the particular body type.

Summary of Automatic Body Functions

The body works pretty well by itself. It is a social order of 100 trillion cells, organized with many different functions arranged to act together as one unit for maintaining a balanced internal environment that supports life. Each cell benefits from the health of other cells, which is why it is impossible to have a healthy body if one part of the body is ill. The reciprocal arrangement of all the systems of the body means that when one system's automatic functions are impaired, the rest of the systems will begin to malfunction as well. As a result, all cells begin to suffer – with eventual dysfunction and cellular degeneration. An extreme dysfunction leads to death of the organism.

Chapter 6

THE DIGESTIVE PRINCIPLE

The digestive principle is simply this: *what we take in we become*. What we can digest becomes our strength, what we can't digest becomes our weakness. The weakness shows itself in the form of symptoms and illness.

In simplest terms, the foods that create our life are proteins, carbohydrates, and fats. Digestion is the process by which proteins, carbohydrates, and fats are broken down. Since we cannot absorb them into our system directly, they must be reduced to bite-size, edible chunks. Once broken down we can take them into the body. We call this process *absorption*. If they cannot be broken down, they are useless for our bodies and may contribute to ill health through the formation of a toxic residue (ama). In Ayurvedic teaching, disease results from the accumulation of ama, particularly degenerative diseases. The Ayurvedic therapy program to help remove this accumulation is called *pancha karma*, meaning "five actions." Pancha karma is a complete five- to seven-day Ayurvedic cleansing and rejuvenation program with a tradition that goes back five thousand years. If patients needed cleansing five thousand years ago, they must *surely* need it more now with the pollution of our air and water and the level of pesticides and herbicides in our food supply. See the Resource Guide at the back of this book for a listing of pancha karma therapists.

The Role of Digestion in Good Health

The basic purpose of the gastrointestinal tract is to give the body water, nutrients, and electrolytes. To do this it has to be able to 1) move food through the system, 2) digest the food with enzyme secretions, 3) absorb what has been digested, 4) distribute the nutrients to the blood for transport to the cell, and 5) eliminate the waste products of digestion.

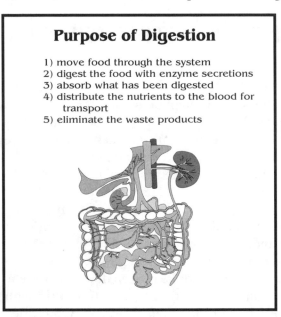

Purpose of Digestion

1) move food through the system
2) digest the food with enzyme secretions
3) absorb what has been digested
4) distribute the nutrients to the blood for transport
5) eliminate the waste products

The simplest route of food through the digestive tract would look like this: Food is taken into the mouth and chewed, which breaks the particles into smaller, more manageable pieces. As this occurs, the salivary glands secrete an enzyme called *ptyalin* that begins to digest sugar. After swallowing, the food passes through the esophagus to the stomach where *HCL* (hydrochloric acid) is secreted to begin digesting protein. *Pepsin* is secreted to further digest protein. The food is mixed with the enzymes and passed into the small intestine where pancreatic enzymes begin to break the food into smaller and smaller pieces. These pieces are broken into units small enough to pass through the walls of the small intestine into the blood. The blood then distributes the nutrients to the rest of the body. The remaining undigested bulk material is passed into the colon and eliminated.

Digestion, then, is about taking big things and making them smaller so they can fit into our blood stream and eventually into our cells. Enzymes are chemicals in our digestive tract that break the proteins, carbohydrates, and fats into the smaller and smaller chunks necessary for absorption. All food is made up of proteins, carbohydrates, and fats. What, then, are proteins, carbohydrates and fats made up of?

Proteins consist of amino acids linked together (peptide linkages). Digestion of protein involves breaking down the big, long chains of amino acids into smaller and smaller chains so they can get into the system.

Carbohydrates consist of glucose molecules linked together. Starch is a long-chain carbohydrate made up of many glucose molecules linked together. The larger molecules are broken into smaller ones and eventually into a single molecule of glucose that we can absorb into the blood stream.

Fats consist of fatty acids and glycerol (triglycerides). Fat is digested when the fatty acids and the glycerol are separated so absorption into the blood can occur.

Digestion Vs. Metabolism

Digestion is the mechanical and chemical breakdown of food into simple molecules that the body can absorb and deliver to the cells. What then happens in the cells is called *metabolism*. Metabolism is the physical and chemical change that takes place within a cell that makes it possible to continue living. In other words, the cell takes what digestion and absorption deliver and changes it into something edible by the cell; this is metabolism.

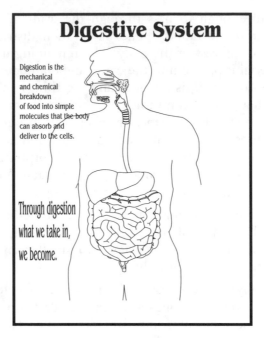

Digestive System

Digestion is the mechanical and chemical breakdown of food into simple molecules that the body can absorb and deliver to the cells.

Through digestion what we take in, we become.

Proteins, carbohydrates, and fats are energy foods that can be oxidized in the cell. This process then releases large amounts of energy that become available for various physiological functions. We require energy for every body activity from muscle contraction to hormone secretion. In other words, the cells burn glucose and use the energy released to keep themselves functioning and well fed.

What does food do for us?

Food is simply the carrier of the raw material needed by our cells to keep them functioning and healthy. Ideally, food we consume should be of good quality and fully digested (broken down into the smallest fragments possible) for total absorption. "Bad stuff" like beer and pizza should occupy a very small, or nonexistent, place in our diet. But of course that is the ideal, and that is rare.

Are there good and bad foods?

What is good for one person may not be good for another, even if it says so in the most prestigious books and publications. I myself ate soy products for most of my 25 years as a vegetarian. Though soy products are good food for many people, they weren't for me, because I had developed an allergy to soy. Allergies can develop due to improper digestion of a particular food. What isn't broken down in digestion can become toxic to our system. Because I was unable to properly digest and absorb soy products, my continued intake of this food stressed my body, resulting in symptoms of chronic fatigue. Some people may develop symptoms of headache, neck or back pain, nausea, etc. from eating certain foods. Others may have difficulty breathing.

By the way, when I stopped eating all soy products the fatigue went away and didn't return (unless I ate something with soy in it).

Food allergies and/or food sensitivities are the result of the body's inability to process what we have taken in. Even if the food we eat is supposed to be good for us, we can still have a negative reaction to it. From the Ayurvedic body-type approach, what is good for a Vata may not be good for a Kapha.

Is there a right diet for everyone?

The answer is yes. There *is* a right diet for everyone. However, there is no *one* right diet for everyone. Some bodies simply have more difficulty digesting certain types of foods than others. Some are allergic or intolerant to certain food groups such as dairy, meat, or grains. *There is no one-diet-fits-all*. We have, however, a way to determine which diet and foods are best based on our ability to digest proteins, carbohydrates, and fats.

Is there a simple program to make us healthy?

Simple? No. A little complicated, yes. It is complicated

because we are not used to thinking this way. Once we get beyond a few unfamiliar words – like Vata, Pitta, and Kapha; ectomorph, endomorph, and mesomorph – most of us can understand and follow this approach quite easily. The approach is the Body Type Zone Program – a specific set of principles and practices for each body type; a Vata Body Type Program, a Pitta Program, etc. Each set of practices helps to nurture the body with daily healthful practices.

If we follow a Body Type Zone program, will we be healthy? Maybe, or it might just make us healthier than we were. Either way, these programs are based on the needs of our particular body type, so we will be heading in the right direction.

Understanding the Digestive Principle

The digestive principle is knowing what we can easily digest. To find out what we can digest, we must look at our genetic makeup. For example, a Vata (Metabolic Type I) has less ability to digest protein than a Pitta (Metabolic Type II) or Kapha (Metabolic Type III); therefore the Vata Zone Diet has a different ratio of proteins to carbohydrates to fats than the Pitta or Kapha Zone Diet.

The percentage of protein, carbohydrates, and fats we can easily metabolize will change according to our body type or body type imbalance. A Vata will eat less protein but need to augment its ability to digest and absorb it. A Pitta will eat less fat but needs to augment his or her enzymes to digest what fat it does take in. A Kapha will need to decrease sugar consumption and increase the ability to handle sugar and starch. Once we know what we can and cannot digest, we can change what we take into our systems. The questionnaires in Chapter 13 will help you discover your body type.

Chapter 7

DIGESTION AND HEALTH

The Breaking of Bonds: Enzyme Function

Chapter 6 outlined the basic purpose of digestion which is to (1) move food through the system, (2) digest the food with enzyme secretions, (3) absorb what has been digested, (4) distribute the nutrients to the blood for transport to the cell, and (5) eliminate the waste products. Now we will look further into the process of breaking down each of the major food components and what can go wrong in the process of digestion.

Digestion of Protein

We cannot live without protein. Proteins are major dietary components made up of many amino acids linked together in various ways. The characteristics, shape, and linkage of the different amino acids give them their physical and chemical properties.

$$H_2N - \underset{\underset{R}{|}}{\overset{\overset{H}{|}}{C}} - C \underset{OH}{\overset{O}{\diagup}}$$

Amino Acid

Protein Digestion in the Stomach

When food enters the stomach and distends its walls, special cells of the stomach called *parietal* cells secrete hydrochloric acid (HCL). This drops the resting pH from the norm of 5-6 to a range of 2-3 – very acid. HCL reduces pepsinogen to *pepsin*, which allows the enzyme (pepsin) to begin the process of breaking down the long-chain amino acids into shorter and shorter chains. Pepsin will not work in a pH range above five; therefore, if there is a problem with hydrochloric acid production, the level of protein digestion will drop (the Vata Effect – reducing and constricting).

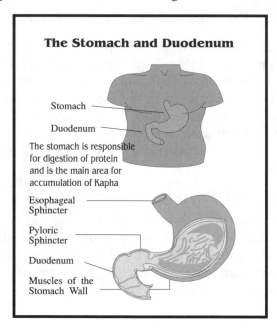

The Stomach and Duodenum

Stomach

Duodenum

The stomach is responsible for digestion of protein and is the main area for accumulation of Kapha

Esophageal Sphincter

Pyloric Sphincter

Duodenum

Muscles of the Stomach Wall

Proteins are made up of amino acids hooked together:

A.A. + A.A. + A.A. + A.A.

To digest amino acids so the body can use them, they must be separated. Pepsin in the presence of H2O (water) splits the amino acid bonds, leaving two separate amino acids, one with an attached hydrogen (H) molecule and one with an attached hydroxyl (OH) molecule. This makes amino acids available for cellular metabolism.

A.A.+ A.A./pepsin /H2O = A.A. with (H) and A.A. with (OH)

Another important action of pepsin is its ability to digest collagen, a major component of animal tissue. No other enzyme can do this; therefore, if we are deficient in pepsin production, we will not digest protein completely. Because people who suffer from deficient pepsin production may have problems digesting protein and meat, they are natural vegetarians. Again, according to Ayurveda, incomplete digestion (a Vata Effect) is a major cause of disease.

A most important concept emerges when we begin to understand that we may eat enough protein but may not be able to digest it, based on the level of enzyme production available. "You are what you eat" doesn't exactly apply then, does it? *You are what you can digest.* What we can't digest ends up as toxins in the body, making us sick. In the Ayurvedic tradition disease is a result of incomplete digestion, not simply intake.

Pepsin begins the process of digestion by breaking bigger chunks of food into smaller ones. Most of the digestion of protein occurs in the small intestines. The larger proteins, when acted upon by pepsin, are split into proteoses, peptones, and polypeptides. These are then split further by the enzymes trypsin, chymotrypsin, carboxpolypeptidase, and proelastase into polypeptides and amino acids, which the enzyme pepti dase further acts upon to split into amino acids.

These big words and run-on sentences may put you to sleep! The point is that the stomach has its role in protein digestion and so do the small intestines. We completely digest only a small portion of protein in the center of the small intestines, however. The micro-villi, in the brush border of the walls of the intestines, have within them enzymes that finally split dipeptidase into amino acids. According to Guyten, 99 percent of the final products of protein digestion are absorbed as amino acids; however, a few larger macro-molecules of peptides and whole proteins are absorbed. Again, according to Guyton " . . . even these very few molecules of protein can sometimes cause serious allergic or immunological disturbances." Ayurveda also teaches that undigested food particles (ama) cause serious allergic and immunological disturbances.

Digestion of Fat

Fats and oils are a big part of our life. We need a little background to understand how they differ and why we digest them differently. At room temperature, fats are solid and oils are liquid, because the molecules of each are arranged differently. Fats and oils are made up of three (tri) fatty acid molecules bonded or attached to one glycerol molecule.

FA + FA + FA + GLY

When in this form we call them *triglycerides*. These are building blocks for cell structure, and function as precursors for other chemicals in the body such as prostaglandins, which we require for the brain cells, adrenal glands, and testes to function. The structure or shape of a molecule determines its behavior in our bodies, making some fats capable of healing (unsaturated fats) and some of killing (saturated fats).

The fatty part of the fatty acid chain is made up of carbon and hydrogen atoms bonded together, which are water-hating (hydrophobic), corresponding to Vata, which is dry. The acid part of fatty acids is water loving (hydrophilic), corresponding to Kapha, which is moist, wet. This structure gives fatty acids their different qualities of action. Fatty acids' different lengths further change their behavior in the body for good or bad. The shorter/smaller the chain of fatty acid, the easier it is to digest, because it is less taxing on our liver than the longer-chain fatty acids. Short-chain fatty acids provide calories, energy, and heat. Short-chain saturated fatty acids (SaFAs) help construct cellular membranes, but are also stored as fat. They are found primarily in butter and milkfat.

Long-chain saturated fatty acids (SaFA's) tend to be sticky and clump together, causing a tendency to blood clots, cardiovascular disease, diabetes, and clogged arteries. They are found in meats such as beef, mutton, and pork.

According to Udo Erasmus in his book *Fats that Heal, Fats that Kill*, deficiencies in certain fatty acids (Linoleic Acid - LA) can produce loss of hair, excessive water loss, drying up of glands, sterility in males, miscarriages, and arthritis-like conditions – which are also the result of the Vata Effect. Deficiencies in Alpha-Linolenic Acid (LNA) can produce high blood pressure, sticky platelets, tissue inflammation, and edema, which are also the result of the Kapha Effect.

Linoleic acid (LA), a polyunsaturated fat belonging to the W6 family of fatty acids, is found in safflower, sunflower, hemp. soybean, walnut, pumpkin, sesame, and flax. Alpha-Linolenic Acid (LNA) belongs to the W3 family of fatty acids, which Udo Erasmus refers to as superunsaturated fats. LNA is found in canola, soy, flax, hemp seed, bean, walnut and dark-green leaves.

Erasmus further states:

> "Our body uses unsaturated and essential fatty acids to construct membranes, create electrical potential, and move electrical currents. It can also burn them to produce energy . . .
>
> ". . . The resulting highly unsaturated molecules serve functions in all cells, and are especially key in the most active tissues of our body: the brain, sense organs, adrenal glands, and testes."

In Ayurveda, fats are one of the main therapies for decreasing the Vata Effect, which is associated with the electrical systems of the body.

When we eat fat, where is the fat supposed to go? What is it supposed to do when it gets there? Let's follow some food fat through our digestive system.

When we eat fatty food, very little digests in the mouth.

[7]Erasmus, Udo; *Fats that Heal, Fats that Kill*; Alive Books, Burnaby BC Canada 1986,1993

We swallow the chewed food and it goes into the stomach where protein is digested, but little fat. Fat does not digest well in the acid environment of the stomach, but passes through to the more alkaline environment of the small intestines, where it is broken down more readily. From the stomach the food passes into the first part of the small intestine (*the duodenum*) where the fat begins to emulsify. Fat can take awhile to digest (the intestines can digest only about 10 grams of fat per hour) which is why, when we've eaten a lot of fat, we feel like we have a slow, sluggish digestive system.

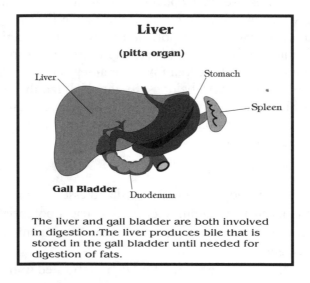

Liver

(pitta organ)

Liver
Stomach
Spleen
Gall Bladder Duodenum

The liver and gall bladder are both involved in digestion. The liver produces bile that is stored in the gall bladder until needed for digestion of fats.

Fat digestion takes place in several stages, the first as food is mixed with bile as it enters the small intestines. As we have said, bile is a product of the liver, made of cholesterol, and stored and concentrated in the gall bladder. When fat is present, the gall bladder empties bile into the small intestines to break down the fat into smaller pieces. (If we have our gall bladder removed, our digestion will change, as we need bile to digest fat.) The intestinal lining cannot assimilate fatty foods. The enzyme at the end of the fat digestion cycle (the pancreatic enzyme lipase) is not able to break down the big fat globules efficiently; however, bile breaks the globules into tiny droplets so the lipase can act on them. We call this process emulsification. Emulsification speeds up the rate at which fatty material is digested by increasing the surface area of the fat exposed to the enzyme lipase.

Digestion of Carbohydrates

The normal diet contains three major sources of carbohydrates: sucrose (shorter chain simple sugars), lactose (milk sugar), and maltose. Carbohydrates are made up of simple sugars (glucose molecules) connected in various ways. A simple sugar, or monosaccharide, is one glucose molecule; disaccharides have two glucose molecules; polysaccharides have many glucose molecules linked together. Sucrose is a disaccharide made of glucose and fructose joined. In our diet, this is most familiar to us as cane sugar. Lactose is a disaccharide sugar found in milk. Maltose is a disaccharide, found primarily in beer. Starches are the most complex sugars, called polysaccharides, which have many sugars connected. They are most present in grains and most non-animal food.

> Sucrose = fructose and glucose
> Lactose = galactose and glucose
> Maltose = glucose and glucose

The body accepts only glucose as a fuel. Only glucose can get into the cell to be used for energy; everything else must be broken down to glucose. As we chew our food, an enzyme called *ptyalin* is secreted from the parotid glands in the mouth to begin the process of carbohydrate digestion. Ptyalin breaks down starch, a polysaccharide, into the smaller two sugars (disaccharides). Remember that digestion is about breaking things down into smaller pieces. In this case, the hooked-together glucose molecules need to be separated to be used by the cells. The polysaccharide isn't broken down in just one step, however; there are several intermediate steps between a polysaccharide (many sugars) and the monosaccharide (simple sugar) which can be used by the body.

Starches, when acted upon by the pancreatic enzyme *amylase*, are broken down into maltose – a shorter length (3-9) sugar. Maltose, in the presence of the enzyme *maltase* then becomes glucose (simple sugar). Lactose, or milk sugar, in the presence of the enzyme *lactase* becomes *galactose* and glucose. Sucrose, in the presence of the enzyme sucrase become fructose and glucose.

Getting glucose into our cells is not as easy as one, two, three. Enough enzymes must be present at every level to ensure proper and complete digestion. For thousands of years, Ayurveda has recognized the need for enzyme stimulation and good digestion. In theory there is always enough enzyme formation. In reality our enzyme levels are not sufficient to break down many food components properly. We can attribute this to overeating foods that require more processing, thus putting a strain on our body's ability to produce the needed enzymes. Aging and diseases are other factors in the body's inability to produce sufficient enzymes. Also, our modern diet has become deficient in the nutrients needed to supply our body's ability to create the enzymes or stimulate the organs that produce them.

We actually digest only about 5% of the carbohydrate portion of food in the mouth. This may be because food isn't in there long enough; therefore, chewing our food well is the first, most important, and simplest action to improve our health. If we gulp our food down it will not be properly digested, and according to Ayurveda, we can trace most diseases to just this.

When we swallow food it passes through the esophagus into the upper part of the stomach where carbohydrate digestion continues for another bit before stomach secretions are mixed with the food. Then, because stomach secretions are acid in nature, the pH range drops very low, making the sugar enzyme ptyalin inactive and unable to break down the carbohydrates.

We digest refined starches such as white flour, white rice, pasta, or enriched white flour more rapidly, so they are more likely to be turned into fat than the more complex carbohydrates such as whole wheat flour or whole grain brown rice. Carbohydrates such as sugar are digested rapidly by the body, so all simple sugar can quickly turn to fat.

How Sugar Becomes Fat

When we want to understand the body type diets and our ideal "Zone," we need to understand how sugar turns into fat. A Vata type can eat many carbohydrates without seeming to gain weight. A Kapha type gains weight just looking at a cookie. This has do with the levels of insulin, glucagon, somatostatin and thyroid hormones in the body, discussed in Chapter 9.

When the food we eat gets to the stomach and passes into the small intestines, we call it chyme. It no longer resembles what we ate. It's all mixed up with enzymes and other foodstuffs. As the chyme passes into the small intestines, the pancreatic enzyme amylase further acts upon the carbohydrates.

We digest starches (carbohydrates) within 15-30 minutes after they enter the first part of the small intestine (the duodenum). They are then converted into maltose and other smaller sugars. The walls of the small intestines have small *villi*, which are finger-like protrusions that secrete enzymes. These four enzymes – lactase, sucrase, maltase and dextrinase – can break down lactose, sucrose, maltose, and other small sugars into monosaccharides, or simple sugars. These simple sugars can then be used by the cells.

Summary

Remember that the goal of digestion is to break all food down to a simple sugar, the monosaccharide glucose. This final product of the digestion of starches, or polysaccharides, can be absorbed into the bloodstream and taken to the cells.

Chapter 8

BODY TYPES AND DIGESTION

According to Ayurveda, we can trace most disease processes back to a disturbance in the digestive system. Perhaps the most important Ayurvedic concept for Westerners is the strength of the digestive fire called *agni*. Agni is not real fire, of course, but the digestive fire that breaks the chemical bonds in our foods, making them smaller to allow vital elements and nutrients to pass through our digestive system into our cells. When the digestive system is not functioning properly, the cells receive no raw materials, and eventually the organism fails to thrive. *Therefore, the prime directive of the body is to fulfill the need of every cell for energy derived from protein, carbohydrates, and fats.*

Four Levels of Digestive Fire

1. **Balanced:** Digestive fire that creates the most perfect health is neither too much nor too little. A good, regular appetite marks a balanced digestive fire. Complete digestion feels comfortable, with no gas, constipation, or bloating. Bowel movements are regular, energy is abundant, and the senses are clear. Each body type can experience this balanced digestive fire.

2. **Irregular or Fluctuating:** Digestive fire that is on and off leads to an inability to digest food completely,

resulting in mal-absorption, nutritional deficiencies, gas, constipation, and bloating. The appetite fluctuates from very hungry to very little desire for food. The out-of-balance Vata usually has an irregular digestive fire.

3. **Excess or High:** Digestive fire that is too "hot" also results in an inability to digest food completely. The appetite can be excessive, causing overeating, which further results in undigested food. Vital nutrients are not digested or absorbed by the body when the digestive fire is too hot, powerful, and abundant. The out-of-balance Pitta may have an excessive digestive fire.

4. **Diminished or Low:** Digestive fire that burns regularly at a lower temperature similarly results in incomplete digestion. This is a slow-burn digestive fire that never quite gets chemically "hot" enough to do the job. The appetite may be low as well. A Kapha type often has low digestive fire.

Vata Digestion

In Ayurvedic teachings the Vata type has the weakest and most irregular digestive system. Sometimes it works well and sometimes it doesn't. A Vata's appetite may also be very irregular, swinging from one extreme to another. One question I ask when I am determining body type is "Have you ever forgotten to eat?" A Vata will often answer yes to this question because their appetite just isn't strong. A Pitta with a good appetite will look at me as though I am crazy and say "Of course not." Kaphas with a low appetite may also answer no simply because they have a watch – they know when it is time to eat.

Vata's increased sympathetic nervous system stimulation and somatostatin hormone release reduces and constricts the body's digestive abilities. Therefore the Vata type has more difficulty digesting food in general and protein in specific, requiring that they pay more attention to eating habits that recognize Vata's need for regularity. This irregular digestive capacity of Vata leads to inconsistent and diminished nutrients absorbed into the system, contributing to Vata's tendency toward a slender, even "gaunt" body type. Vata can eat a great deal without gaining weight or putting on much muscle. As proteins may be most difficult for the Vata to digest, a vegetarian diet offers a much more comfortable eating experience without the gas and bloating Vatas otherwise experience. Because of the ease of digestion it is possible that vegetarians are predominantly Vata body types (and vegetarians in general tend to be thinner).

Pitta Digestion

According to Ayurveda, Pitta has the hottest and most powerful digestion. Usually Pitta has the best appetite, and when hungry, must eat. They rarely forget a meal. They simply cannot. They will eat larger amounts of food than a Vata or a Kapha and if healthy, will burn it up. If their digestive fire is too high, however, they may be unable to process the nutrients they take in.

Pitta's increase in both the sympathetic and parasympathetic nervous systems and glucagon hormone release results in a strong digestive capacity, but a tendency to become overactive – thereby affecting Pitta's ability to metabolize fat completely. Excess dietary fat may be the hardest for the Pitta to digest. When eaten in excess, fats cannot be emulsified and associated problems with the gall bladder and liver may arise, along with a tendency to gain weight. Excessive digestive fire also results in symptoms of heartburn, gastritis, and colitis. We may take an antacid to reduce the fire, but though this may help in the short term it only complicates the digestive problem by not treating the cause – an excess of digestive fire.

Kapha Digestion

In Ayurvedic tradition, the Kapha has the slowest but the most efficient digestion. The Kapha seems to eat less and gain more, a result of the most thorough digestion of food.

Those with weight problems know instinctively that there are variances in the metabolism of different people. They can eat less than other, thinner, people but they still seem to gain and gain. This is the metabolism of the Kapha. Kapha's general increase in parasympathetic nervous system stimulation increases its ability to digest food, but also results in a slow, sluggish digestive system. Since the food passes through the system at a slower rate, more thorough absorption occurs. This results in the well-fed Kapha body.

The Kapha also has an increased insulin response to carbohydrates, causing the tendency to gain weight and requiring a diet that reduces carbohydrates. A reduced-carbohydrate diet will also lessen the stress to the pancreas.

Stages of Digestion

Stage I—The Kapha Stage

The Kapha stage begins in the mouth with the salivary enzyme amylase beginning the process. The food then moves into the stomach, which is lined with heavy mucous (a Kapha quality) that protects it from the action of the very potent hydrochloric acid and other enzymes necessary for the breakdown of food. In this stage food becomes more liquid (also Kapha) and uniform in consistency so further digestion can take place. Symptom imbalances in Kapha, such as lack of appetite, low or slow digestion and nausea, result from eating too many heavy, sweet, oily foods – all Kapha in nature.

Stage II—The Pitta Stage

The Pitta, or second, stage of digestion occurs in the small intestines. Here is where bile (Pitta) is secreted from the gall bladder and other digestive enzymes such as protease, lipase, and carbohydrylase are secreted from the pancreas and small intestinal wall. These serve to break down the chemical bonds of protein, carbohydrates, and fats in our food. This is the main stage of digestion where heat (Pitta) and energy are released into our body.

Problems occurring with this stage relate to an increased digestive fire that may result in heartburn, gastritis, and ulcers. Hot and spicy foods aggravate these symptoms.

Stage III—The Vata Stage

Vata governs the third stage of digestion. According to Ayurveda, the large intestine is the seat of Vata. Here water and other elements are extracted (Vata) from food and re-circulated in the bloodstream to be cleansed by the liver. We will eliminate what remains through normal bowel movements. Symptoms such as constipation and gas are common with a Vata imbalance.

Ama, the Toxic Load

When the digestive fire doesn't burn and metabolize the food mass sufficiently, there remains undigested material that becomes a poison in the body. In Ayurvedic teaching, this undigested material (Ama) can and does become a toxin in the system by creating dysfunction in cellular metabolism. Remember that each cell has an intracellular fluid that must have an exchange of nutrients and waste for it to survive. Ama is like a film of grime that settles in and around the cell. With sufficient accumulation of this toxic load, the cell's particular function is then hindered and eventually shuts down. According to Ayurveda, a poison, if properly digested, will not create illness; but even the highest quality food, if not digested properly, will become a poison that can make us sick.

Dr. David Frawley, author of *Ayurvedic Healing*[8] writes: "When agni is sufficient there will be no toxic build ups in the body, the mind and senses will be clear and acute, and we will possess the energy to change our lives in a positive direction. When agni is deranged we will suffer from dullness, heaviness, stagnation and cloudiness of emotion and perception."

[8]Frawley, David; Ayurvedic Healing; Passage Press, Salt Lake City, Utah

Chapter 9

METABOLIC ZONE OF VATA, PITTA, AND KAPHA

We are not all blessed with the same digestive system. What works for one will not necessarily work for all. Our ability to metabolize food depends entirely on what kind of digestive machine we have. Good wholesome food, if not properly digested, can and does create illness. We are created anew every day. Every time we sit down to a meal, we have the opportunity to enhance or undermine our health. Food is the ultimate drug. The proper food for us, properly digested, will make us whole. Our overall health, our ideal weight, emotional stability, mental acuity, and general well-being depend on what we can and cannot digest. That simple.

For each body type there exists an ideal ratio of protein to carbohydrates to fats. Our health will improve or deteriorate depending on the percentage of each component we consume. In *The Zone*, Barry Sears suggests a ratio of protein to carbohydrates to fats necessary for the individual who has problems with weight gain. His research led him to conclude that increased carbohydrate consumption causes an increased insulin hormone secretion and a corresponding decreased glucagon hormone secretion, which results in weight gain. Overweight people (often Kapha types) do not necessarily have a problem with dietary fat consumption, *but may have a problem with dietary carbohydrates turning to fat.*

Barry Sears also states that not all people who eat carbohydrates will have this negative insulin hormone reaction.
Research by Gerald Reaven at Stanford University [1987]
suggests that there is a genetic component to this phenome-
non. His research shows there are three different insulin
responses to carbohydrate consumption. Twenty-five percent
of the population shows an increased insulin response to carbohydrates while another 25% shows none. The remaining
50% are somewhere in the middle of this continuum. In
Ayurveda, the genetic component is called your inherited
constitution, or body type.

The three insulin responses to carbohydrates:

> 25% decreased insulin response
> 50% varied response
> 25% increased insulin response

Those who have little or no increased insulin response
may eat large amounts of carbohydrates and gain little weight
(the Vata body type.) Those who show an increased insulin
response may gain weight easily (the Kapha body type), and
the group in the middle, with a variable response to carbohydrate consumption, may or may not gain weight (the Pitta
body type).

The Zone points out that increased carbohydrate consumption in general will cause weight gain and other related
problems. A strong correlation exits between the individual
with an increased insulin response to carbohydrate consumption and the Ayurvedic description of the Kapha: they both
gain weight as a result of eating carbohydrates. Though he
didn't call it such, Barry Sears described the physiology of the
Kapha.

If a proper ratio of carbohydrates to fats to proteins
exists for the Kapha body type, a proper ratio for the Pitta
and Vata must also exist and they must be different from one
another. The idea that one body type is able to digest some
macro nutrients better than another suggests a proper ratio of

macro nutrients for each type. When we combine the extensive study of body types with modern scientific research and principles of physiology, we conclude that there may indeed be a Zone for Metabolic Type I (Vata), for Metabolic Type II (Pitta), and for Metabolic Type III (Kapha).

Just What is The Zone?

According to Barry Sears, ". . . simply put it's the metabolic state in which the body works at peak efficiency . . . in the zone you'll enjoy optimal body function: freedom from hunger, greater energy and physical performance, as well as improved mental focus and productivity." He further states " . . . fatigue and listlessness are replaced by feelings of energy and high competence, weight loss ongoing, life in the zone creates considerable health benefits." About health care he writes, " . . . being in the zone can become the basis for a new kind of low cost yet ultra-effective healthcare reform: a reform in which the individual takes charge of his or her own body, and keeps that body in a state of exquisite good health."

This all sounded very familiar. Ayurveda also describes increased health and vitality to be found when we follow the program recommended for our body type. Being in the Vata Zone, for example, would mean that we would meet the metabolic requirements of optimal health for a Vata body type – not only the macro nutrient ratio requirements such as protein, carbohydrate and fat, but the micro nutrients as well, such as vitamins, minerals, enzymes, and trace elements. The elements that create a healthy Vata are different than those that create a healthy Pitta or Kapha. Therefore, the Zone for each type will be different.

My definition of the Zone is *that special metabolic state unique to a person's genetic constitution where the body functions at optimal efficiency, the tissues and organs function at their highest level, and the mind, will, and emotions are balanced with perfect tension to the pursuit of their destiny.*

Benefits of Living in the "Zone"

The benefit of living in the Zone is the amplification of the positive characteristics of our body type, with a resulting beneficial effect on our physiology and our health.

A Healthy Vata

A Vata type is healthiest living in the zone of balanced Vata physiology. Vata Effect tends toward a faster metabolic rate and catabolism (tissue reducing and constricting). Vatas have a smaller, thinner, yet graceful frame. Their limbs tend to be long and sleek. Vatas are very tireless and animated with great energy and vitality. Their digestion is delicate and discriminating. They experience a precise and defined mental nature. A healthy Vata's eyes reflect modest enthusiasm. Their life force is animated, affording them great activity levels. They have a vibrant manner marked by graciousness and enthusiasm. Vatas have the energy to accomplish most anything they desire.

A Healthy Pitta

A Pitta type is healthiest living in the zone of balanced Pitta physiology. Pitta Effect tends toward a more powerful metabolism (tissue transformation and modification). Pittas have a medium frame with well-developed muscles that excel in athletic ability. Their digestion is strong and complete. Their appetite for food, and for life, is great. They experience a bold and commanding sensual nature. Their rosy skin and healthy complexion show the fire of their hearts. A Pitta's eyes are penetrating and show total comprehension. Their immune system is powerful and efficient. They have a commanding and authoritative manner marked by compassion and good judgement. They have the courage to accomplish most anything they desire.

A Healthy Kapha

A Kapha type is healthiest living in the zone of balanced Kapha physiology. Kapha Effect tends toward a slower metabolic rate and anabolism (tissue building and expanding). Kaphas have a large but firm musculature with strong bones and joints. They have well-proportioned bodies with great endurance and stability. Their digestion is strong with good absorption. They have a strong and powerful sensual nature. Their skin is soft and smooth with a healthy, light complexion. A healthy Kapha's eyes are large, attractive, and calming to the rest of the world. Their hair is very thick, plentiful and beautiful. They have a strong immune system, affording them great health. They have an intelligent, thoughtful manner marked by calm and clarity of intent. They have the patience to accomplish most anything they desire.

The Vata Body Type and Protein Metabolism

Why is protein metabolism a problem for a Vata type? Generally speaking, proteins, in anyone's diet, are the hardest to break down. Remember that the Vata has the least ability to process food overall. More Vatas may be vegetarians than any other body type simply because they have difficulty with protein digestion – they can't easily eat meat. Therefore, when Vatas are imbalanced, they may need to reduce their consumption of meat (protein) to return to health.

The Pitta Body Type and Fat Metabolism

According to Ayurveda, the Pitta type has difficulty with fat metabolism. The liver makes bile and stores it in the gallbladder to emulsify fat (break it down into smaller molecules). In a Pitta, bile and other digestive enzymes are produced in excess, creating an overabundance of heat – resulting in symptoms such as heartburn, gastritis or colitis. When Pittas are imbalanced they may need to reduce their dietary fat to reduce stress on enzyme production capacity, which allows them to return to health. Also, according to Ayurveda, the sweet taste is beneficial to the Pitta, suggesting that carbohydrate consumption is not as damaging for them as it is for the Kapha.

The Kapha Body Type and Carbohydrate Metabolism

According to Ayurveda, the Kapha type has the most difficulty metabolizing sugar. The pancreas, a Kapha organ, controls sugar metabolism by secreting insulin. When we consume too many carbohydrates the physiological reaction is increased insulin secretion. Therefore, when Kaphas are out of balance they will need to reduce carbohydrate consumption (sugars, starches, etc.) to return to health.

Earlier in my life I was working as a musician in a fancy oriental restaurant. The owner, a small Chinese man, and I had many opportunities to chat about what it meant to be a vegetarian. One day he said to me "Denny, I am puzzled. Why aren't you skinny like most of the veggies I know?" Well at the time I didn't have a clue. Though I had lost quite a bit of weight and was at my ideal weight for my height, I was not skinny. I did not fit the "veggie" profile; no matter what I did, I did not fit that profile. I have never been a slight man – I have a great tendency to go the other way, which is part of my Kapha nature.

I increased the grains in my diet to follow the conventional wisdom at the time. I continued, however, to gain weight even with a vegetarian diet. When I began to gain, I just ate more grains – which was the wrong thing to do for my Kapha body. But I didn't know that at the time.

Summary

The *body type zone* is based on the differing abilities of each type to digest protein, carbohydrates, and fats. Vatas need help balancing protein metabolism; Pittas need help balancing fat metabolism; Kaphas need help balancing carbohydrate metabolism. According to Ayurveda, the overall ability of Vata to digest almost anything is impaired compared with Pitta or Kapha. Pitta has the best and hottest digestive capacity; Kapha has the slowest and possibly the most efficient. *To get to and stay in our healthy zone, we need to realize what we can and can't digest.* To do this we need to know our body type, our genetic makeup.

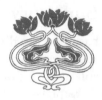

Chapter 10

HORMONES AND DIGESTION

The Zone of health for each body type is based on the ability of the body to digest proteins, carbohydrates, and fats, and the body's levels of insulin, glucagon, somatostatin, and thyroid hormones in response to the stresses in life.

Pancreatic Hormones

The pancreas is an organ involved in the formation and secretion of the enzymes needed to digest protein, carbohydrates and fat. It is made up of two parts, the Acini, which secretes digestive enzymes into the small intestines, and the Islets of Langerhan, which secretes insulin, glucagon, and somatostatin—three very important hormones—directly into the blood.

The Islets of Langerhan are further made up of three types of cells: alpha, beta, and delta cells. Alpha cells secrete glucagon; beta cells secrete insulin; delta cells secrete somatostatin. All three hormones have different but reciprocally-related functions. For example, insulin secretion inhibits glucagon, while somatostatin inhibits both glucagon and insulin.

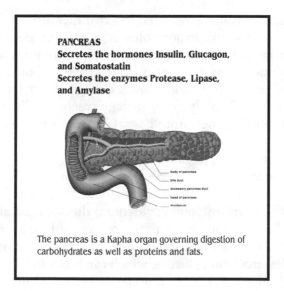

PANCREAS
Secretes the hormones Insulin, Glucagon, and Somatostatin
Secretes the enzymes Protease, Lipase, and Amylase

body of pancreas
bile duct
accessory pancreas duct
head of pancreas
duodenum

The pancreas is a Kapha organ governing digestion of carbohydrates as well as proteins and fats.

Insulin

When insulin is secreted into the blood, it travels to other cells to make them more permeable to the glucose that is floating in the blood. Remember, carbohydrates are broken down into smaller and smaller molecules until only glucose remains. Glucose can't get into the cells of the body without some help, and insulin essentially opens the door to the cells so glucose can get in. Once in, glucose enters into cellular metabolism by becoming the fuel and energy for running the cell.

Insulin and the Physiology of Kapha

Kapha Effect of Increased Insulin on Carbohydrate Metabolism

The pancreas is responsible for controlling sugar metabolism through insulin secretion. In Ayurveda the pancreas is a Kapha-associated organ. Guyten's *Textbook of Medical Physiology* states "Insulin is a hormone associated with energy abundance, when there is great abundance of energy-giving foods in the diet, especially excess amounts of carbohydrates and proteins, insulin is secreted in great quantity."

One of insulin's major roles is storing excess carbohy-drates as fat (adipose tissue). When we consume too many carbohydrates, insulin secretion causes the carbohydrates to be stored in the liver and muscles as glycogen (an energy reserve unit). When glycogen storage reaches its limit, excess carbohydrates are then stored as fat. So sugar is stored as fat. Too many complex carbohydrates, no matter how "good for you," are stored as fat. According to Ayurveda, even rice and grains, in excess, can convert to fat and cause weight gain.

To summarize the Kapha Effect: after a meal high in car-bohydrates, from any source, glucose is digested and absorbed into the blood, which triggers the release of insulin from the pancreas. This causes the doors of the body's cells to open and take in the circulating glucose, which can result in further stor-age as glycogen and fat in muscle, adipose, and liver tissues. Insulin also causes dietary fat to be stored as adipose tissue.

Kapha Effect of Increased Insulin on Fat Metabolism

Though not as important in the short term, insulin has a strong long-term effect on the body through its role in fat metabolism. Insulin increases the use of glucose by the body's tissues, while decreasing the use of fat. That means that stored fat will stay in storage. Insulin also promotes fatty acid synthesis, resulting in more fat stored. According to Guyten, ". . . this is especially true when more carbohydrates are ingested than can be used for immediate energy, thus provid-ing the substrate for fat synthesis." In other words, when we eat more than our body can immediately use, the body has to store it – and we gain weight. Especially Kaphas. Some Pittas will also gain weight, but as Vatas do not experience the increased insulin level associated with sugar consumption, they also do not experience the associated weight gain.

Kapha Effect of Increased Insulin on Protein Metabolism

Insulin is not only active in the storage of carbohydrates

and fats, but proteins as well. It actively increases the amino acid transport into the cells, which increases the formation of proteins. We describe this effect as an *anabolic* process – which means the building up of tissue. Anabolism is a Kapha trait, accounting for the larger, heavier body structure.

Increased Insulin and Body Weight

In almost all cases increased insulin response causes weight gain, a Kapha Effect.

Insulin and Vata

Vata Effect of Decreased Insulin on Protein Metabolism

Vatas have a lower insulin secretion level, which can cause protein depletion. Protein storage comes to a halt and the body begins to use proteins stored in muscle and organ tissue. We call this metabolic breakdown of tissue *catabolism*, a Vata trait. Vatas, therefore, are usually smaller and thinner.

Vata Effect of Decreased Insulin on Fat Metabolism

When insulin secretion is minimal the mechanisms for use of fat for energy are increased. In other words, stored fat is now on the top of the list for conversion to energy. Most of the effects of increased insulin noted above are reversed. Important to note is the activation of the hormone-sensitive enzyme lipase, which is found in the fat cells, causing release of stored triglycerides into the blood as fatty acids and glycerol. This becomes the primary available energy source. A long-term deficiency of insulin is associated with atherosclerosis, heart attacks, and strokes.

Decreased Insulin and Body Weight

In many cases, decreased insulin response causes a decrease in weight gain, a Vata Effect.

Summary

Insulin promotes the use of carbohydrates for energy and suppresses the use of fats for energy. The lack of insulin causes more fat use. Insulin secretion is entirely controlled by the level of glucose in the blood. When glucose concentration is low, insulin secretion is also low, causing fat to be used as the energy source. When the glucose level is high, insulin secretion is also high, and carbohydrates are used as the main energy source. Insulin levels, then, control whether fats or carbohydrates will be used as fuel for the body. An increase in insulin is associated with the physiology of Kapha. Decreased insulin is associated with the physiology of Vata.

Glucagon

Glucagon and the Physiology of Pitta

Pitta Effect of Increased Glucagon on Carbohydrate Metabolism

The Pitta body type has a lowered insulin response to carbohydrate ingestion and an increase in glucagon secretion. Glucagon is the hormone secreted by the alpha cells of the pancreas. Its main actions and effects are somewhat opposite to that of insulin. When blood glucose concentration is low, glucagon secretions act to increase it (the body does not like low blood sugar). Glucagon raises the glucose level by affecting the liver's stores of *glycogen*, which are the energy reserve unit. The liver changes this glycogen into useable glucose released into the blood in a process called *glycogenolysis* (the breakdown of glycogen). This reserve can last for a few hours but will eventually become depleted.

Glucagon is associated with the physiology of Pitta. Ayurveda teaches that the sweet taste (and carbohydrates in general) decrease Pitta. Therefore, glucagon secretion decreases Pitta.

Pitta Effect of Increased Glucagon on Protein Metabolism

Another effect of glucagon is *gluconeogenesis*. This is the formation of new glucose from stimulation of liver functions that result in increased use of amino acids by the body. These amino acids are then converted into glucose. High concen-

trations of amino acids from a high protein meal will cause increased glucagon secretion. This increases glucose concentrations by stimulating the liver conversion of amino acids to glucose, which puts fuel on the fire (the Pitta Effect).

Pitta Effect of Increased Glucagon on Fat Metabolism

Another effect of glucagon is the activation of adipose cell lipase, making fatty acids available for conversion to energy, another aspect of Pitta physiology. In other words, stored fat is mobilized as an energy source. Glucagon also strengthens the heart and increases bile secretion, a Pitta Effect (the Sanskrit word Pitta means bile). Exercise also causes increased glucagon secretions which results in the shift to stored fat as fuel source.

Increased Glucagon and Body Weight

In most cases, increased glucagon secretions will result in a medium body build. If the Pitta does gain weight it is most likely to be a result of problems with fat metabolism.

Importance of Blood Glucose Regulation

The most important factor in controlling glucagon and insulin secretions is blood glucose concentration. When blood glucose concentration is low, glucagon kicks in, causing a return to normal levels. When high, insulin kicks in to return it to normal levels. Why is this so important? Because we require a constant level of glucose in the blood stream to supply the brain adequately. The brain runs on glucose. Therefore the prime directive of metabolism is to get glucose to the cells, and ultimately to the brain.

Somatostatin/Thyroid Hormone

Somatostatin / Thyroid Hormone and the Physiology of Vata

Somatostatin is secreted by the delta cells of the Islets of Langerhans in the pancreas. According to Guyten, ". . . almost all factors related to the ingestion of food stimulate somatostatin secretion. They include (1) increased blood glucose,

(2) increased amino acids, (3) increased fatty acids, and increased concentrations of several gastrointestinal hormones released from the upper gastrointestinal tract in response to food intake."

Somatostatin secretion has many consequences, most of them decreasing the Vata Effect. Somatostatin acts with the Islets themselves to inhibit insulin and glucagon secretion. It reduces the movement and action of the stomach, the small intestines, and the gallbladder, resulting in digestive distress and constipation often experienced by the Vata type. Somatostatin also reduces both secretion and absorption in the gastrointestinal tract, which are all actions of the physiology of Vata.

The **thyroid** gland is found just below the larynx. It secretes two very significant hormones, thyroxine (T3), and triodothyronine (T4). These hormones increase the rate of a metabolism, the Vata Effect. Guyten states " . . . the rate of utilization of foods for energy is greatly accelerated. Although the rate of protein synthesis is increased, at the same time the rate of protein catabolism is also increased, the mental processes are excited, and the activity of most of the endocrine glands is increased."

Effects of Thyroid Hormones on Carbohydrate Metabolism

The thyroid hormones stimulate all aspects of carbohydrate metabolism, including increased cellular uptake, increased formation of glucose (gluconeogenesis), increased breakdown of glycogen in the liver (glycolysis), and increased absorption from the small intestines. These increases in metabolism are associated with an increase in Pitta and Vata Effects.

Effects of Thyroid Hormone on Fat Metabolism

All aspects of fat metabolism are also enhanced with thyroid hormone stimulation, causing stored fat to be used as an energy source at a higher rate than usual. This is a Vata physiology effect, which results in a body with little fat storage.

Thyroid Hormone and Body Weight

In most cases, increased thyroid hormones and increased somatostatin secretions cause decreased body weight, a Vata characteristic.

Both somatostatin and thyroid hormones increase the Vata Effect, somatostatin by decreasing the action of the functions of the digestive organs, thyroid hormones by increasing the rate of utilization of carbohydrates, proteins and fats. Both these characteristics cause increased Vata and decreased body weight.

Adrenal Hormones

Adrenal Hormones and the Physiology of Kapha

Above each kidney lie the adrenal glands. The adrenal glands are composed of two separate parts, the adrenal medulla and the adrenal cortex. The central part of the adrenal gland is the medulla, which is functionally related to the sympathetic nervous system. The medulla secretes the hormones epinephrine and norepinephrine when the sympathetic nervous system is stimulated. These two hormones are then carried to all tissues of the body. Their effect on the tissues is almost identical to that resulting from stimulation of the sympathetic nervous system. This effect, however, lasts five to ten times longer because the hormones are removed from the blood more slowly.

As does direct sympathetic stimulation, norepinephrine causes inhibition of the gastrointestinal tract, constriction of the blood vessels, increased heart activity, and dilation of the pupils. Epinephrine causes the same symptoms but has a greater effect on the heart and lesser effect on the constriction of the blood vessels. Also, epinephrine has a greater metabolic effect on the overall metabolism of the body. These are both similar to the Vata and Pitta Effect.

Kapha Effect of Cortisol Secretion

The adrenal cortex secretes a different set of hormones called *corticosteroids*, which are manufactured from cholesterol. These hormones have slightly different shapes, giving them different functions in the body. We call the two major types of corticosteroids mineralcorticoids and glucocorticoids.

Mineralcorticoids regulate the potassium concentration in the extracellular fluid in relation to sodium and chloride concentrations. The mineralcorticoids are said to be the life-saving portion of the adrenals when an imbalance in these concentrations arises. Glucocorticoids, of which cortisol (hydrocortisone) is one, affect the metabolism of protein, carbohydrate, and fat in response to stress. When excess sympathetic stimulation has depleted the body the next step is replenishing and building up of tissue, the Kapha Effect. Cortisol stimulates carbohydrate metabolism and gluconeogenisis. Cortisol also decreases the protein stores in the body converted to glucose. When a great excess of cortisol exists in the body, the muscle systems can become so weak that walking without exhaustion is difficult. The immune system also becomes depleted.

In the same manner that cortisol stimulates carbohydrate and protein metabolisms it also promotes mobilization of fatty acids from the adipose or fat stores in the body. This does not, however, offset the increased weight gain associated with increased cortisol secretion, a major Kapha Effect.

Almost any types of stress, ranging from trauma, infection, surgery, heat or cold, to mental or emotional pressure will cause an increase in the level of cortisol secretion, which is associated with the calming Kapha Effect. Its effects are anti-inflammatory as well.

Summary

By examining the characteristics of the physiology of Vata, Pitta, and Kapha and comparing them with the actions of the hormones involved in blood glucose regulation, we can conclude that the three basic body types produce different levels of hormone secretion resulting in different levels of metabolic actions in the body.

Hormones and Body Type Response

The Vata Body Type

It is obvious that each body type has a unique level of hormone response. Of the three, the Vata body type has the lowest insulin response to carbohydrates and a greater increase in somatostatin and thyroid secretion. These hormones serve to decrease both glucagon and insulin levels, creating the highest catabolic state (tissue breakdown) of all three types, and resulting in the thinner, leaner Vata body.

The Pitta Body Type

The Pitta body type has a lowered insulin response to carbohydrate ingestion and an increase in glucagon secretion, which results in increased fatty acid mobilization from stored fat, leading to a body that is leaner than the Kapha but not as lean as the Vata.

The Kapha Body Type

The Kapha body type has a greater insulin response to carbohydrate ingestion. Therefore, we see the more negative side effects of increased insulin concentrations in the Kapha, such as weight gain. The Kapha tends to have a lower level of thyroid hormone secretion, resulting in a sluggish or slower metabolism.

Chapter 11

WEIGHT CONTROL AND YOUR BODY TYPE ZONE

Weight gain for many people is an enormous problem, especially in a culture that puts so much emphasis on being slender. We diet, exercise, and even fast to keep our weight down. We try every new fad, every new theory to help us become slim and stay slim. From the point of view of Ayurveda, however, not everyone could be or even *should* be slender.

Several years ago, I had a patient who was a definite Kapha body type. She was rather tall, not thin but certainly not fat, and very beautiful. However, she was unhappy because she was what she described as a "Vata wanna be." She wanted to be skinny. No matter what she did, no matter how much she exercised, no matter what diet she tried, skinny was never to be found. Her inner nature was Kapha, but she did not appreciate it very much. She had beauty, curves and a nice full figure, but she wasn't slender. It took her awhile to understand that not all slender women are beautiful and that her gifts were her own. It made me realize that a basic requirement for happiness is understanding and appreciating our own inner nature.

Of the three body types, Kapha has the heaviest frame and the biggest problem with weight control. As pointed out in other chapters, this relates to hormone regulation, protein, carbohydrate, and fat consumption, and the strong genetic tendency of the Kapha body type to increase in weight. The Pitta type can gain unwanted weight if they have strong secondary Kapha traits and consume too many fats. The Vata body type seems to stay slim no matter what they do.

Weight Loss and Weight Control

There are only two problems associated with weight. Too much or too little. Either way, it can be a health problem, though being too thin in this country is much more acceptable than being too heavy. When we think of weight control, most people think of losing unwanted pounds. In fact some people may actually need to *gain* weight. Generally, Kaphas don't have much sympathy for this condition though it certainly can be a significant problem. Obesity, however, can be very serious. It can lead to the development of other disorders such as fatigue, back and leg pain, shortness of breath, sluggishness, lethargy, heart disease, high blood pressure, arthritis, liver problems and other symptoms associated with obesity (Kapha-type symptoms).

Weight Control by Body Type

Ratios of Macronutrients by Body Type

Each body type requires a different ratio of the macronutrients protein, carbohydrates, and fats, to fuel its particular genetic makeup (insulin response, glucagon response, somatostatin response). The percentage is based on what can and can't be digested. As we have noted, when we consume macronutrients that we can't digest they become toxins that can lead to illness.

The proper ratios of protein to carbohydrate to fat (pro/carb/fat) stimulate the appropriate level of hormone response, putting us in the healthy "zone" for our body type. Barry Sears describes the perfect food ratio as 30% protein, 40% carbohydrate, and 30% fat. His entire theory is based on the idea that we eat too many carbohydrates, and that the trend in the last few years toward higher consumption of carbohydrates has not increased our general level of health. In fact, for the Kapha type specifically, this trend has been detrimental. This theory is profound for those of us (Kaphas) who have never understood why we could not keep off the excess pounds when we thought we were eating according to recommended healthy diets.

I would like to take this theory one step farther. When out of balance, a Vata (Metabolic Type I) has difficulty digesting protein; a Pitta (Metabolic Type II) has difficulty digesting fat; a Kapha (Metabolic Type III) has difficulty digesting carbohydrates. Therefore, healthy ratios *for each of the three body types* would look more like this:

Healthy Ratios of Protein/Carbohydrate/Fat for each Body Type Zone			
	Protein	Carbohydrate	Fat
Vata/ Metabolic Type I 20/40/40	20%	40%	40%
Pitta/ Metabolic Type II 30/50/20	30%	50%	20%
Kapha/ Metabolic Type III 30/40/30	30%	40%	30%

To remain healthy and within the optimum range of body weight, Vata, Pitta and Kapha require quite different ratios of macronutrients. What makes a Vata healthy is different from what makes a Pitta or Kapha healthy. Thousands of years of practicing Ayurvedic medicine have led to clearly-defined health programs for each body type, which include recommendations for diet and lifestyle to put you and keep you in your special Zone. In Chapter 14 we will go into the diet and lifestyle plan for each body type based on the above ratios.

Kapha Weight Control

Unwanted weight gain and the inability to lose weight often indicate a Kapha body type or a Kapha imbalance. If we are overweight, chances are we are in a Kapha condition and need to follow a Kapha program – at least for a while. The Kapha program in Chapter 14 is designed to reduce Kapha tendencies and increase Vata and Pitta, allowing us to lose unwanted weight and find our balance. A Vata-kapha (Vk) who has gained weight would follow a Kapha program to reduce Kapha and increase Vata and Pitta. A Pitta-kapha (Pk) who has gained weight would follow a Kapha program. It is all intended to reduce the Kapha imbalance, which is the primary causal factor in weight gain.

A Kapha gains weight through diet and lifestyle practices that increase Kapha tendencies. An immense piece of the weight-loss puzzle is knowing that an increase in carbohydrate consumption (even 'good' complex carbohydrates such as brown rice) will cause increased insulin production and lead to weight gain. Again, Kaphas have an increased insulin response to carbohydrates, which sets up the entire metabolic sequence for *deposit* of fat rather than fat utilization. This process is fully described in Chapter 9.

Pitta Weight Control

The Pitta type can gain weight with an overabundance of fat in their diet, as the Pitta body type has difficulty with fat metabolism associated with the liver and gall bladder. This fat consumption without full metabolism will, of course, tend to create weight gain. Pittas can greatly benefit from a Kapha program for weight loss, as it includes carbohydrate reduction as well as dietary fat reduction. When a healthy weight level for the Pitta is achieved, we recommend a switch to the Pitta program.

Vata Weight Control

Because the very nature of Vata is light, it is more unusual for the Vata type to gain weight, but it can happen. A Vata-kapha (Vk) will gain weight, but is usually able to lose it more readily than the Pitta or Kapha due to the speed of the Vata metabolism. Underweight is of far more concern to the Vata. Since Vatas have such a problem with protein metabolism and digestion in general, they need a program that nurtures the body in all ways. The Vata needs to follow the Vata Program in Chapter 14, which is all about nurturing.

Digestive Fire and Weight by Body Type

Digestive fire is our capacity to break down food into usable nutrients for cellular metabolism. This process is described more fully in Chapters 6 and 7. The digestive fire is reflected in our appetite. Simply put, we need to have a good appetite to enkindle the proper digestive fire. The Kapha's digestive fire is lower than a Pitta's, though more regular than a Vata's. Following the Kapha program in general will help increase the appetite and improve the sluggish Kapha digestion. I know that having little appetite seems ideal for someone who is trying to lose weight, but the truth is that excess weight gain is a symptom of an unhealthy imbalance in our system. Restoring a good appetite is part of restoring a vital, balanced, fully functioning, healthy system.

Kapha Type Digestion: As the Kapha digestion is slow and sluggish, more nutrients and calories are absorbed into the body, creating the larger, more nourished system.

Amylase and carbohydralase are the enzymes needed for sugar metabolism and the Kapha body type.

Pitta Type Digestion: The digestive fire of the Pitta is usually strong but when imbalanced may experience difficulty with fat metabolism associated with a deficiency of the enzymes lipase and bile.

Vata Type Digestion: The digestive fire of the Vata is usually much more irregular, sometimes strong and sometimes weak, which may result in an undernourished body. Digestive enzymes such as protease, lipase, and amylase may be helpful in increasing the nutrition level of the Vata.

Lifestyle Therapeutics For Obesity

Kapha-Reducing Plan

No matter what our body type, if we are overweight we need to follow a Kapha-reducing program to slim down. Kaphas especially need to be aware that they will always have a natural tendency toward increasing Kapha. It's too bad if our body type is Kapha and we are Vata wanna-be's, but it is the way it is. If we are a Kapha body type and our weight is under control, we still need to follow the Kapha dietary recommendations in Chapter 14 to keep in balance and keep from re-gaining.

All diets that reduce sugar and fat are Kapha-reducing diets. All exercise programs are Kapha-reducing. All dietary supplements that stimulate fat metabolism are Kapha-reducing. Anything that is Spartan in nature is Kapha-reducing. Kaphas generally don't like it, but it's the way they are made. If we need to lose a greater amount of weight, we can follow the Kapha program much more stringently. The Kapha Program in all its aspects promotes full circle healing (see Chapter 2). If we follow the entire program regularly, it can be of great help.

Herbs and Supplements

Dr. Vasant Lad and Dr. David Frawley described many traditional Ayurvedic herbs as well as many Chinese and Western herbs in their book *The Yoga of Herbs*[9]. Herbs, vitamins, minerals, enzymes and any other supplements beneficial to the metabolism of our body type are important as an adjunct to the body type zone program; however, we cannot lose weight just by taking a pill.

Certain herbs increase Vata while decreasing Pitta or Kapha; some increase Kapha and decrease Pitta, etc. We can classify any substance with an action that we can measure as Vata-, Pitta-, or Kapha-reducing. Kaphas can use herbs and supplements such as haritaki, amalaki, bibhitake, gentian, ginger, gotu kola, and guggul, which increase carbohydrate metabolism and reduce Kapha. Pittas can use herbs such as aloe, dandelion, burdock, red clover, and barberry to improve fat metabolism and reduce Pitta. Vatas can use herbs such as ashwagandha, comfrey root, ginseng, ginger, garlic, and brahmi to increase protein metabolism and reduce Vata.

Kapha-reducing herbs: haritaki, amalaki, bibhitake, gentian, ginger, gotu kola, guggul.
Pitta-reducing herbs: aloe, dandelion, burdock, red clover, barberry.
Vata-reducing herbs: ashwagandha, comfrey root, ginseng, ginger, garlic, brahmi.

Diet: The Kapha-reducing diet program is outlined in Chapter 14. Follow it closely.

Exercise: Kaphas generally hate exercise. Given that, the best exercise for reducing Kapha is one that gets the heart pumping and the body sweating. Aerobic exercise is best for this purpose. If we are Kapha, or suffering from a Kapha imbalance, we need to find something that heats us up and keeps us going for quite awhile. We will feel much better, though we might not admit it.

---

[9]Lad, Dr. Vasant, Dr. David Frawley; *The Yoga of Herbs*; Lotus Light Publishing, Wisconsin 1986

Stress Management: Reduce chaos in your life. Reduce stress in your life. Reduce Vata in your life. Chaos, stress, and nervous tension are not good for any body type. A Vata imbalance in a Kapha can increase the nervous desire to eat – causing, of course, weight gain.

Use the following four indexes to apply the principles of weight control to your life. These indexes are a general guide as to what increases or decreases Kapha. They are valuable tools for understanding what is good and not so good in our diet.

Glycemic and Taste Index

We can categorize foods by the speed at which they enter the blood stream after eating. We call this the glycemic index. Foods with a faster rate of entry have a higher glycemic index and those with a slower rate of entry have a lower glycemic index. The higher the index, the greater the insulin response and subsequent Kapha Effect weight-gain patterns. Barry Sears' book, *The Zone*, amply describes the relationship of increased weight gain to a diet high in foods with a higher glycemic index. Ayurveda has done this as well. In Ayurveda, the glycemic index is referred to as the "taste of sweet" in the diet.

According to Ayurveda, six taste indexes can be used to monitor the increase or decrease of the Kapha Effect on our physiology. They are: sweet, salty, sour, pungent, bitter, and astringent. The tastes that increase Kapha are sweet, salty, and sour. Therefore, reducing these tastes in our diet will help to reduce the Kapha Effect on our physiology. We don't have to be a Kapha body type to experience the Kapha Effect, of course. If we are having trouble with weight gain, no matter what our body type, reducing these tastes will help reduce the Kapha Effect on our physiology.

Tastes of Food	
Sweet	Sugar, honey, molasses, milk, certain grains (rice, barley, wheat, buckwheat, cornmeal, millet, rye, amaranth, quinoa), sweet fruits (apples, berries, pears, grapes, sweet melons, figs), sweet vegetables (corn, carrots, onions, sweet potatoes)
Salty	Salt, meat, soy sauce, miso
Sour	Lemons, limes, cheese, yogurt, vinegar, some fruits are both sweet & sour (strawberries, cantaloupe, grapes, oranges, pineapple, papaya, rhubarb), tomatoes
Pungent	Cayenne pepper, chili peppers, onions, garlic, ginger, bell peppers, carrots
Bitter	Greens (collard, kale), endive, romaine lettuce, spinach, tumeric
Astringent	Beans, lentils, aduki beans, black beans, chickpeas, mung dhal, pinto beans, soy beans, navy beans, cabbage, broccoli, cauliflower, potatoes, celery, green beans, artichoke, lettuce, potatoes, spinach, squash, carrots, corn

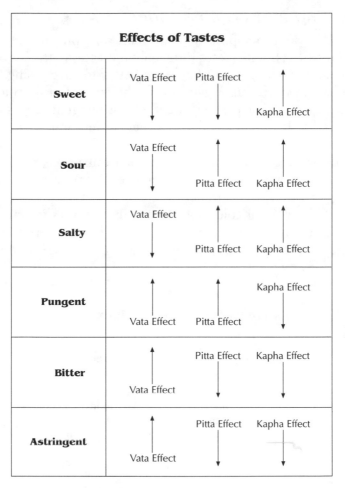

Effects of Tastes			
Sweet	Vata Effect ↓	Pitta Effect ↓	Kapha Effect ↑
Sour	Vata Effect ↓	Pitta Effect ↑	Kapha Effect ↑
Salty	Vata Effect ↓	Pitta Effect ↑	Kapha Effect ↑
Pungent	Vata Effect ↑	Pitta Effect ↑	Kapha Effect ↓
Bitter	Vata Effect ↑	Pitta Effect ↓	Kapha Effect ↓
Astringent	Vata Effect ↑	Pitta Effect ↓	Kapha Effect ↓

Notice that what increases the Kapha Effect (sweet, sour, salty) decreases the Vata Effect, and what decreases the Kapha Effect (pungent, bitter, astringent) increases the Vata Effect. According to Ayurveda, foods that increase the glycemic index, as well as foods that are sour and salty, increase the Kapha Effect. To reduce the Kapha Effect on your physiology and help control unwanted weight gain, eat a diet high in the foods listed in the Kapha Zone Program.

Heating and Cooling Index

We can also approach weight control from the view of temperature: hot increases Pitta, cold increases both Vata and Kapha. Therefore, warm foods are better for decreasing the Kapha Effect of weight gain. From the view of taste, cold is bitter, then astringent, then sweet. Hot is pungent, then sour, then salty. In the chart above, sweet, bitter, and astringent decrease Pitta, and pungent, sour, and salty increase Pitta. When we are Kapha or have a Kapha imbalance, we want generally to increase our biological fire (Pitta) by consuming pungent, bitter and astringent foods.

By decreasing cold foods in our diet such as ice cream, iced soft drinks, ice water, etc. we can decrease the Kapha Effect. And for your information, heating up ice cream doesn't work very well.

Increase/Decrease Kapha Effect	
Increase	**Decrease**
Oily, moist foods, such as: milk, cheese, butter, ghee, cooking oil, fried foods	**Dry foods**, such as: dried fruits, granola, breads, crackers, millet, barley
Sweet foods, such as: carbohydrates, sugars and grains	**Pungent foods**, such as: cayenne, chilies, ginger, onions
Heavy foods, such as: most meats	**Light foods**, such as: salads, soups, fruits, vegetables

Dry and Moist Index

We can classify tastes as dry or moist as well. Sweet is wettest, then salty, then sour. Pungent is driest, then bitter, then astringent. Again, if we look at the qualities of Kapha, the water element, we notice it is the most moist. Sweet foods increase that moisture (the Kapha Effect) by increasing the water element. Oily foods increase the Kapha Effect. Dry foods decrease the Kapha Effect.

Heavy and Light Index

We may also classify foods as heavy or light. Heavier foods such as meat and grains are generally oilier and harder to digest. Some examples of heavier (oiler) grains are rice and wheat. Lighter foods such as soups, salads and vegetables are easier to digest. How much food we take into the body is also important: the larger the amount, the heavier the index; the lesser amount, the lower the index. The quality of heavy is Kapha; the quality of light is Vata. Therefore to decrease Kapha, we must increase lightness in our diet by eating smaller amounts and eating foods that are easy to digest. This is the basis of the Kapha Zone Program.

The Colorado Holistic Center Ayurvedic Weight Loss Program

The digestive fire is at it's strongest level between 10:00 A.M. and 2:00 P.M. Traditional Ayurveda suggests the biggest meal of the day should be consumed at lunch because this is when the body is able to digest the most food without the formation of ama, the toxic load associated with disease. To lose weight, we can take advantage of this increase in the digestive metabolic fire by taking in a smaller meal than normal such as a brothy soup or a balanced protein/fat/carbohydrate meal replacement drink with the appropriate herbs and spices that further reduce Kapha (see resources section). Though replacing a meal with a protein drink is not the traditional Ayurvedic approach, it is effective if used in accordance with the full program. As well, eating this light meal does fall into the general category of "decrease Kapha".

We find on this program the patients appetite starts to return in a real way. This is a good sign that the physiology is changing. The evidence of a good appetite is indication of better health. The following meal at dinner should be a Kapha decreasing meal. You will probably be hungry by the time dinner comes around. Eating earlier is better than eating later. Don't eat later than 7:00 p.m. as this will tend to slow down your digestion. A menu of steamed vegetables, a little grain, perhaps a little fish, the appropriate spices for taste and interest and you have your meal.

This program may be followed for 1-2 months with proper supervision. To find a qualified ayurvedic counselor see our resource guide.

Staying in Your Zone

Staying in the Kapha Zone

An increase in the Glycemic/Sweet Index increases Kapha, so
decrease sweet foods

An increase in the Cooling Index increases Kapha, so
increase 'hot' foods

An increase in the Wet Index increases Kapha, so
decrease moist foods, increase dryer foods

An increase in the Heavy Index increases Kapha, so
decrease heavy foods, increase lighter foods

Staying in the Pitta Zone

An increase in the Pungent Taste Index increases Pitta, so
decrease pungent foods

An increase in the Heating Index increases Pitta, so
decrease 'hot' foods

An increase in the Heavy Index increases Pitta, so
decrease heavy foods, increase lighter foods

An increase in the Moist Index increases Pitta, so
decrease moist foods, increase dryer foods

Staying in the Vata Zone

An increase in the Astringent Taste Index increases Vata, so
decrease astringent foods

An increase in the Cooling Index increases Vata, so
decrease cold foods, increase warm foods

An increase in the Lightness Index increases Vata, so
decrease light foods, increase heavier foods

An increase in the Dryness Index increases Vata, so
decrease dry foods, increase moist foods

Three Patient Profiles:
Weight Control/Weight Loss

J.M. was an overweight man of 28, a Kapha-pitta with a serious Kapha imbalance. He had been overweight almost his entire life. As a child he was "husky." As an adult, he was 50 to 60 lbs. overweight. J.M. began the Kapha program in early April. Though he did not follow the program perfectly, he was successful in losing about 40 lbs. over the next four to five months. Since the Kapha program includes many different practices along with diet, he will be able to continue his weight control as part of a lifelong program of optimum health. As a Kapha he will always need to be on the Kapha program, but will need to follow the program more stringently when he finds himself gaining weight.

H.D. is a 36-year-old female. She had experienced weight gain, lethargy, fatigue, back pain, and menstrual irregularities for several years. She is a Pitta-kapha with a Kapha imbalance. In February she attended my lecture on Ayurveda and came to my clinic for help. After examination, I recommended a temporary Kapha program for her. Although by birth she was a Pitta-kapha, her weight gain put her in the Kapha category. She had gained weight due to problems with fat metabolism, and continued to do so until she began her Kapha program in earnest. She went through pancha karma treatments and diligently applied herself to her regime. After several months she came into my office for another matter (exposure to chemicals). She had lost 30 lbs. and was looking quite healthy. I modified her program to continue her weight loss and to begin a more balanced Pitta-kapha program. When she reaches her ideal weight, she will make a transition to the Pitta program while continuing to be vigilant about weight gain. Currently she is doing just fine. Should she fall off her program and begin to put on weight, she will know how to lose it when she wants.

T.R. was a 64-year-old woman experiencing chronic

fatigue, neck pain, and upper abdominal pain. She also suffered from insomnia and restlessness. She was a Vata-pitta with an extreme Vata imbalance. Clinically she had a hyperthyroid condition that increased her metabolism and made her very thin. For her condition I recommended pancha karma and also a Vata Program. She followed the program very well and gained several pounds as a result of eating the Vata diet, the most nourishing of all three diets. By following the rest of the Vata program she reduced her fatigue and neck pain and almost eliminated her abdominal pain. If she continues to follow the program, she will continue to receive lifelong benefits.

Summary

Weight control is a health problem for many people. Losing or gaining weight can be nearly impossible until we understand the special metabolic furnace associated with our body type. Barry Sears' book, *The Zone*, indicates a proper ratio of protein to carbohydrates to fats necessary for weight control and better health. This ground-breaking research has gone a long way to diffuse the popular myth of weight loss resulting from diets high in carbohydrates.

Kaphas gain weight due to their increased insulin response to carbohydrates; Pittas gain weight due to problems with fat metabolism; Vatas have trouble gaining weight at all. Reducing carbohydrates in the diet and following the Kapha Zone Program accomplishes weight control for a Kapha. Reducing fat in the diet accomplishes weight control for a Pitta. Vatas can gain weight by increasing both the Pitta and Kapha qualities in their diet, both fat and carbohydrates. All metabolic types can benefit by following the Glycemic and Taste Index, the Heating and Cooling Index, the Dry and Moist Index, and the Heavy and Light Index which increase or decrease the qualities necessary to control weight.

Chapter 12

DIAGNOSIS AND BODY TYPE ZONES

Knowing our genetic makeup and understanding our body type brings significant health benefits. The importance of knowing whether we are prone to heart attacks or cancer cannot be overstated. A Vata type *is* genetically different from a Pitta or Kapha. Genetic makeup accounts for the differences in the strength and quality of the digestive system, the immune system, hormone and endocrine secretions as well as every other aspect of physiology.

Purpose of Diagnosis

The basic purpose of diagnosis is to decide the *cause* of disease. For Western medicine, however, diagnosis is often relegated to distinguishing one disease from another. Western medicine likes to try to pin a diagnosis down by naming it. Wholistic medicine sees that as futile because illness rarely has just one cause. More often, it is multi-factorial. From a wholistic point of view, a disease is a name given to a combination of system malfunctions throughout the body. The greater number of systems that no longer work, the greater the likelihood of chronic degenerative disease.

A diagnosis can differ for the same symptoms; i.e., depending on the frequency and duration of a pain in the head, a medical doctor might diagnose migraine; a chiropractor might diagnose a subluxation of the spine; an acupuncturist might diagnose an imbalance of *chi* in the large intestine. All could be right – as we have said, symptoms usually arise from more than one cause. For any one problem there could be many links in the chain of body adaptations to system malfunction. This is what makes diagnosis difficult.

An accurate diagnosis is extremely important. Many different therapies are available, but none should be applied until a working diagnosis is in order. A disease process can get very bad very quickly. It is a waste of time to try different therapies without knowing what they can do for us – and in some cases it is dangerous. If we have a significant health problem, we need to see a doctor or health care practitioner skilled in the art of diagnosing. Preferably it will be someone with training in and understanding of wholistic medicine. At present, few medical doctors practice wholistically. Though today many more chiropractors practice wholistic medicine, the majority choose spinal adjustments as their main therapy. While adjusting the spine is part of a wholistic health regime, it is not the only treatment a patient may require. Naturopaths have trained in "alternative" therapies, but are not licensed to diagnose and are not considered primary care physicians in most states. That leaves a dilemma: how do we help ourselves without endangering ourselves? Perhaps the most obvious choice is to become our own health advocates. By knowing our body type constitution and what therapies and practices are beneficial for that type, we can better control and manage our body for greater health.

How to Help Diagnose Your Condition

Most health care practitioners will use tests to determine the extent of a patient's condition. This is appropriate. However, once obvious disease pathology is ruled out, modern medicine has little to offer patients who suffer from chronic degenerative conditions. Therefore, by helping to diagnose our own condition according to our body type and associated imbalances we can help in our own recovery in a very powerful way. We can learn to find the cause of our symptoms based on the qualities of Vata, Pitta, and Kapha and how they apply to our health.

Reclaiming Your Inner Nature

I like to think of our birth constitution as our true inner nature. As our acquired imbalance becomes stronger, our birth constitution becomes weaker. We don't *lose* our birth constitution, but its qualities become obscured by the stronger qualities of our imbalance. When we set about getting healthy we are really reclaiming our own inner nature, our true self. In the above example, as Kapha increased, Pitta decreased. The biological fire went out, or at least diminished. Some peoples' lives change dramatically when they regain a glimpse of their former selves. If our true inner nature is Pitta (or Vata or Kapha), then that is where our destiny lies.

Summary

The real purpose of diagnosis is to identify the underlying factors that cause disease. We can help this process by finding out the basic constitution, or genetic makeup, of our body and how it has changed over the years. Then, using this information, we can help bring our body back into balance and eliminate dis-ease.

Chapter 13

ANCIENT WAY
BODY/MIND TYPING

Determination of Body Type

Ayurveda actually names seven body types: Vata pitta (Vp), Vata kapha (Vk), Pitta vata (Pv), Pitta kapha (Pk), Kapha vata (Kv), Kapha pitta (Kp), and VataPittaKapha (VPK). We can determine our body type if we know the qualities that make up each type. For instance, one quality of Vata is light. Therefore, if our body is thinner and lighter or if we have more qualities of Vata than anything else, then we are probably a Vata type. If we are heavier and have always had problems with weight gain, we are probably *not* a Vata type. It's as simple as that.

To find your body type fill out the two questionnaires in this chapter. In the first, answer the questions as to how you are now (Acquired Constitutional Imbalance). In the second, answer the questions about how you were when you were young, or when you were healthier (your Birth Constitution). For instance, if you are a 50-year-old male, about 5 foot 10 inches tall, weighing 235 lbs., you may have more Kapha characteristics; but if you weighed only about 170 lbs. when you were a younger man, your original healthy constitution may be more Pitta. Remember, the Pitta type has a medium frame and carries less weight. Therefore, you may have *acquired* a Kapha imbalance over the years (through eating too much ice cream?). I know *I* did.

It is important to know both your Acquired Constitutional Imbalance (Test I) and your Birth Constitution (Test II). Any imbalance between the two can then be addressed with the proper Body Type Zone Program.

Body Type Questionnaire I—
Acquired Constitutional Imbalance

A nswer the following questions by describing yourself as you presently are, as you have been within the last year or so, or since the onset of a recent illness. For example, if you have been suffering from fatigue, insomnia, poor appetite, headaches, or anxiety for the last six months, but not before, answer the questions from the point of view of the last six months. This will help find where your imbalance lies.

0= describes me not at all
1= describes me a little
2= describes me well
3= describes me the most

My hair tends to be:	___fine, dry, curly
My hair color is:	___med. or light brown
The amount of hair is:	___average
My skin tends to be:	___dry, rough, tough
My complexion is:	___darker
I seem to have:	___smaller bones than others
My body is:	___thin, gaining weight is difficult
My level of energy is:	___erratic; up and down
My stamina, ability to carry things to completion is:	___variable; sometimes I go for long periods, other times I accomplish only a few things and I'm finished
I am comfortable with:	___ heat, I don't like cold or wind
My appetite is:	___variable; sometimes I have no interest in food and skip meals, or forget to eat
I like to eat food that is:	___warm, oily, moist
I generally eat:	___quickly, and often eat many small meals

___fine but straight

___wavy, thick, shiny

___blond, reddish, or early gray

___dark brown, black

___thin too early balding

___full, thick

___sensitive, delicate (but I hate to admit it)

___smooth and oily

___more reddish, freckled

___lighter, even pale

___medium-size bones

___larger, longer bones

___medium; sometimes I gain weight, but it's easy to lose

___Heavy, gaining weight is easy (just *think* of food and gain!)

___moderate to high; I find it easy to push myself

___usually pretty good and steady, but it takes awhile to get going.

___very good; I can go for long periods with much intensity; there is always more to accomplish

___excellent; I can out-last most people if I am motivated to do so, but I'd rather be relaxing

___cold; I perspire easily & thrive in winter

___Heat or cold; dislike damp; tolerate extremes well

___excellent; when I am hungry, I need to eat or I get irritated and angry

___good. I can skip a meal, but usually don't

___cool or cold

___warm and dry

___moderately fast

___slowly, but a lot

My sleep is:	___very light; easily interrupted (usually sleep 4-6 hours)
My interest in sex is:	___minimal, unless romance is involved
I am sensitive to:	___loud noises, or chaotic activities
My emotional moods:	___change often & easily; I can respond quickly (or over-respond)
My reaction to stress is:	___fearfulness, anxiety
When it comes to money I:	___am impulsive
I learn:	___very quickly, but often forget
I learn best by:	___listening to a speaker
I can remember:	___best in short term
I speak:	___quickly and precisely, sometimes excessively; with enthusiasm
The positive trait that best describes me is:	___lively
In relationships, I:	___am able to adapt to many different kinds of people & have many friends
Others might describe me as:	___spacy/indecisive

___sound, moderate; (sleep about 6-8 hours)	___very deep; it is hard to wake up; (sleep 8 - 10 hours)
___moderate to strong	___generally very strong
___bright glaring lights	___strong odors
___are intense; I have been called quick-tempered	___are even-tempered; slow to anger, slow to do anything. there's no hurry
___irritation, frustration or anger	___calm and collected
___spend, but usually don't overspend	___tend to save
___quickly	___rather slowly, but I remember
___reading or visual aids	___associating with another memory
___well overall	___long-term very well
___clearly, precisely; I am detailed, well organized	___slowly, deliberately, with moments of silence
___determined	___easygoing, peaceful
___often choose friends on the basis of their values	___am slower to make friends, but am loyal
___intolerant, annoyed	___stubborn, sluggish

Others might wish I were more:	___grounded
Taking this test makes me feel:	___indecisive
I like exercise:	___very much. I like to run, ride bikes
I don't like:	___cold weather
My moods:	___change quickly
I work:	___very quickly, with a lot of initiative
I walk rather:	___quickly
My elimination tends:	___to constipation, infrequent bowel movement
My mental nature is:	___very quick, restless
I get excited:	___easily and often
I become anxious and worried:	___very easily
My digestion is:	___irregular, sometimes good, sometimes not
My memory is:	___short
I react to problems and difficulties in life:	___with anxiety; I tend to be indecisive, I worry

___tolerant, less judgmental

___enthusiastic, involved

___irritated

___bored beyond belief

___very much, and do it with great intensity

___very little; but it makes me feel better

___hot weather

___cool and damp

___change slowly

___are consistent, non-changing

___with moderate speed

___slowly and methodically

___moderately fast but determined

___slowly, steady, with deliberate speed

___to soft or runny stools

___to heavier, well-formed stools

___very sharp, a keen intellect

___calm, steady, and stable

___less easily and less often

___slowly, not easily excited

___occasionally

___rarely

___very good, though sometimes I have heartburn

___slow and sluggish

___medium

___long

___with anger, irritation, and frustration

___with calm; a steady and stable approach

I recognize more of myself in the following healthy attributes and behavior:	___cheerful, enthusiastic, resilient, imaginative, spontaneous, sensitive, exhilarating, friendly, flexible, adaptable, stimulating, alert, life of the party, optimistic, active mind
I recognize more of myself in the following unhealthy attributes and behavior:	___worried, nervous, complaining, anxious, grieving, restless, apathetic, unfocused, depressed, impatient, fearful, insecure, unpredictable, high strung, resisting regularity, over-active mind, quick to burn out, chaotic, spacy, failure to complete projects, difficulty concentrating, insecure
When I see myself as healthy, I generally see myself as being:	___flexible, good communicator, having an acute awareness of the scope of things, knowledgeable, cognizant, active, lively, vital, enterprising, adaptable, enthusiastic, having a good sense of unity, good comprehension, energetic, with a positive attitude, an initiator, with the ability to make changes and move things along.
When I see myself as out of balance, I see myself as being:	___unreliable, having false enthusiasm, untrustworthy, undependable, apprehensive, distressed, disruptive, superficial, nervous, anxious, agitated, restless, disturbed, indecisive

___intelligent, confident, enterprising, joyous, sweet, strong, forceful, practical, fair, just, courageous, exuberant, self-developed, a leader, ambitious, methodical, efficient, adaptable, pleasant, clear-minded, energetic, friendly, fiery

___calm, peaceful, sympathetic, courageous, loving, forgiving, steady, serene, affectionate, stable, quiet, patient, humble, committed, unshakable, generous, compassionate, down-to-earth

___domineering, angry, resentful, hostile, self-criticizing, irritable, impatient, outbursts of temper, argumentative, tyrannical, critical of others, intolerance of others, intolerance of delays, hurtful, hot headed, frustrated

___clinging, possessive, tendency to mother, caring to extremes, manipulative, quiet, withdrawn, hopeless, rigid, unable to accept change, insecure, unwanted, unloved, over attached, procrastinator, passive, greedy, stuck, inflexible, stubborn, stagnant

___a clear thinker, intellectual, rational, bright, intelligent, perceptive, discriminating, warm, friendly, courageous, having leadership qualities, independent, enlightened

___peaceful, content, stable, consistent, loyal, steadfast, firm, faithful, true, constant, nurturing, supportive, calm, loving, forgiving, compassionate, devoted, receptive

___impulsive, ambitious, aggressive, willful, stubborn, critical, dominating, manipulating, angry, proud, vain

___over-attached, greedy, avaricious, covetous, selfish, materialistic, sentimental, wanting comfort and luxury, very controlling

When I see myself as unhealthy, I see myself as being:

___harmful, dishonest, secretive, suicidal, fearful, depressed, self-destructive, addictive

I tend to suffer from the following:

___nervous disorders, backaches, neck pain, headaches. constipation, depression, varicose veins, insomnia, dry skin and wrinkles

I occasionally (or often) experience:

LYMPH (RASA)

___cold hands/feet, dry skin, sunken eyes, numbness or discoloration of skin, psoriasis, eczema, dry cough, anxiety, lack of confidence, insecurity

I occasionally (or often) experience:

BLOOD (RAKTA)

___dizziness, dry eczema, bruises easily, heart palpitations, anemia, heart disease, gout, varicose veins, hypertension

I occasionally (or often) experience:

MUSCLE (MAMSA)

___muscle spasms, muscle atrophy, wasting away, lack of coordination, decreased flexibility, twitching, muscle pain

I occasionally (or often) experience:

FAT (MEDAS)

___dry skin, low backache, cracking of joints, increased thirst, diabetes, wasting away disease

I occasionally (or often) experience:

BONE (ASTHI)

___hair loss, brittle nails, weakening of bone tissue, fractures, bone and joint pain, arthritis, osteoporosis, rheumatoid arthritis, dental caries ___contemptible, paltry, base, hateful, destructive, angry toward others

___peptic/duodenal ulcers, liver disorders, inflammations, fevers, colitis, hypertension, heartburn

___fever, acne, hot flushes, sensitive eyes, criticalness, short temper, increased sweating and thirst, sore throat, psoriasis, eczema, bronchitis

___hot flashes, flushing of skin, burning sensations in hands and feet, inflammation, rashes, nose bleeds, dermatitis

___inflammation of muscles, tendinitis, bursitis, ulcers, gastritis, inflammation of gastrointestinal tract

___profuse sweating, cellulitis, kidney infection, excess urination

___graying hair, early balding, nail infections, burning pain in joints, redness of joints, inflammatory arthritis

___listless, unemotional, dispassionate, unconcerned, apathetic, insensitive, dull, gross, lethargic

___colds, flu, bronchitis, sinus congestion, allergies, diabetes, asthma, sore throat

___water retention, swollen joints, loss of appetite, lethargy, frequent colds, bronchial congestion

___high cholesterol, poor circulation, anemia, gall stones, congestion of liver/bile

___increased nasal mucus, muscle swelling, difficulty moving, rigidity in muscles, lethargy

___high cholesterol, obesity, high triglycerides, fatigue, chronic infections, pancreas and spleen disorders

___swollen joints, bone spurs

I occasionally (or often) experience:

NERVOUS SYSTEM/
MARROW

___dizziness, fainting, lack of coordination, weakening of nervous system, nerve pain, pain and cracking in joints, ringing in ears, tremors, nervousness, insomnia, anxiety, sciatica, neuralgia, feelings of emptiness and fear, loss of memory

I occasionally (or often) experience:

REPRODUCTIVE
(SHUKRA)

___irregular hormonal cycle, painful menstruation, irregular cycle, nervousness, fear, anxiety, low sexual desire, general decrease in vitality

TOTAL: VATA _____

___paralysis, anger, irritability, overly sharp perception, painful perception, neuritis, anemia, dizziness, headache

___dull aching pain, lack of nervous system sensitivity, dullness of senses

___reproductive tissue inflammation, uterine bleeding, painful menstruation, swollen prostate

___enlarged prostate, infertility, impotence, endometriosis, poor resistance to colds and flu, low energy, lack of motivation

PITTA _____

KAPHA _____

Highest Score _____Body type _____

Second Highest _____Body type _____

My acquired (present) body/mind type is:

_____

(Vata-Pitta, Pitta-Vata, Kapha-Pitta, etc.)

Body Type Questionnaire II—
Birth Constitution

The purpose of this questionnaire is to find out more about your true original body/mind type. For example, as you have aged your activity level and metabolism may have changed. Perhaps you have gained some weight, your body begins to look, act, and feel different than it once did. Those pictures in the family album look like another person entirely. Perhaps you are suffering from a Kapha imbalance, causing the weight gain. Or if you have not been well, take the following questionnaire to find out how you responded to life when you were healthy. To find out what your true body/mind type was at birth, take the following questionnaire, answering the questions not as you are now, but as you were at the peak of your health, or at about 20-30 years of age.

If you are under 30 and in very good health, it may be necessary to take only one test.

0= describes me not at all
1= describes me a little
2= describes me well
3= describes me the most

My hair tended to be: ___fine, dry, curly

My hair color was more: ___med. or light brown

The amount of hair was: ___average

My skin tended to be: ___dry, rough, tough

My complexion was: ___darker

I seemed to have: ___smaller bones than others

My body was: ___thin, gaining weight was difficult

My level of energy was: ___erratic; up and down

My stamina, ability to carry things to completion was: ___variable; at times I could go for long periods, other times I accomplished only a few things

I was comfortable with: ___ heat, I didn't like cold or wind

My appetite was: ___variable; sometimes having no interest in food and skipping meals, or forgetting to eat

I liked to eat food that is: ___warm, oily, moist

I generally ate: ___quickly, and often many small meals

My sleep was: ___very light; easily interrupted (usually slept 4-6 hours)

___fine but straight   ___wavy, thick, shiny

___blond, reddish, or early gray   ___dark brown, black

___thin to early balding   ___full, thick

___sensitive, delicate   ___smooth and oily

___more reddish, freckled   ___lighter, even pale

___medium-size bones   ___larger/longer bones

___medium; sometimes I gained weight, but it was easy to lose   ___heavy; gaining weight was easy (just *think* of food and gain!)

___moderate to high   ___usually pretty good and steady

___very good; I could go for long periods with much intensity; always more to accomplish   ___excellent; I could out-last most people if I was motivated to do so, but I'd rather be relaxing

___cold; I perspired easily & thrived in winter   ___ hot or cold temperatures; disliked damp; tolerated extremes well

___excellent; when I was hungry, I needed to eat or would get irritated and angry   ___good. I could skip a meal, but usually didn't

___cool or cold   ___warm and dry

___moderately fast   ___slowly, but a lot

___sound, moderate; (slept about 6-8 hours)   ___very deep; I was hard to wake up; (sleep 8 - 10 hours)

My interest in sex was:	___minimal, unless romance was involved
I was sensitive to:	___loud noises, or chaotic activities
My emotional moods:	___changed often & easily; I could respond quickly (or over-respond)
My reaction to stress was:	___fearfulness, anxiety
When it comes to money I:	___was impulsive
I learned:	___very quickly, but often forgot
I learned best by:	___listening to a speaker
I could remember:	___best in short term
I spoke:	___quickly and precisely, sometimes excessively; with enthusiasm
The positive trait that best described me was:	___lively
In relationships, I:	___was able to adapt to many different kinds of people & have many friends
Others might have described me as:	___spacy/indecisive
Others might wish I were more:	___ grounded

___moderate to strong   ___generally very strong

___bright glaring lights   ___strong odors

___were intense; I have been   ___were even-tempered; slow
called quick-tempered   to anger, slow to do anything –
                                         there's no hurry

___irritation, frustration or   ___calm and collected
anger

___spent, but usually didn't   ___tended to save
overspend

___quickly   ___rather slowly, but I remem-
                                         bered

___reading or visual aids   ___associating with another
                                         memory

___well overall   ___long-term very well

___clearly, precisely; detailed,   ___slowly, deliberately, with
well organized   moments of silence

___determined   ___easygoing, peaceful

___often chose friends on the   ___was slower to make friends,
basis of their values   but was loyal

___intolerant, annoyed   ___stubborn, sluggish

___ tolerant, less judgmental   ___ enthusiastic, involved

If I had taken test then, it would make me feel:	___indecisive
I liked exercise:	___very much. I liked to run, ride bikes
I didn't like:	___cold weather
My moods:	___changed quickly
I worked:	___very quickly, with a lot of initiative
I walked rather:	___quickly
My elimination tended:	___to constipation, infrequent bowel movement
My mental nature was:	___very quick, restless
I got excited:	___easily and often
I became anxious and worried:	___very easily
My digestion was:	___irregular, sometimes good, sometimes not
My memory was:	___short
I reacted to problems and difficulties in life:	___with anxiety; I tended to be indecisive. I worried

___irritated   ___bored beyond belief

___very much, and did it with   ___very little; but it made me
great intensity   feel better

___hot weather   ___cool and damp

___changed slowly   ___were consistent, non-
                                       changing

___with moderate speed   ___slowly and methodically

___moderately fast, but deter-   ___slowly, steady, with deliber-
mined   ate speed

___to soft or runny stools   ___to heavier, well-formed
                                       stools

___ very sharp, a keen intellect   ___ calm, steady, and stable

___less easily and less often   ___slowly, not easily excited

___occasionally   ___rarely

___very good, though some-   ___slow and sluggish
times I had heartburn

___medium   ___ long

___with anger, irritation, and   ___with calm; a steady and sta-
frustration   ble approach

I would recognize more of myself in the following healthy attributes and behavior:

___cheerful, enthusiastic, resilient, imaginative, spontaneous, sensitive, exhilarating, friendly, flexible, adaptable, stimulating, alert, life of the party, optimistic, active mind

I would recognize more of myself in the following unhealthy attributes and behavior:

___worried, nervous, complaining, anxious, grieving, restless, apathetic, unfocused, depressed, impatient, fearful, insecure, unpredictable, high strung, resisting regularity, over-active mind, quick to burn out, chaotic, spacy, failure to complete projects, difficulty concentrating, insecure

TOTAL: VATA _____

___intelligent, confident, enterprising, joyous, sweet, strong, forceful, practical, fair, just, courageous, exuberant, self-developed, a leader, ambitious, methodical, efficient, adaptable, pleasant, clear-minded, energetic, friendly, fiery

___domineering, angry, resentful, hostile, self-criticizing, irritable, impatient, outbursts of temper, argumentative, tyrannical, critical of others, intolerance of others, intolerance of delays, hurtful, hot headed, frustrated

___calm, peaceful, sympathetic, courageous, loving, forgiving, steady, serene, affectionate, stable, quiet, patient, humble, committed, unshakable, generous, compassionate, down-to-earth

___clinging, possessive, tendency to mother, caring to extremes, manipulative, quiet, withdrawn, hopeless, rigid, unable to accept change, insecure, unwanted, unloved, over attached, procrastinator, passive, greedy, stuck, inflexible, stubborn, stagnant

PITTA _____   **KAPHA** _____

Highest Score _____ **Body type** _____

Second Highest _____ **Body type** _____

My birth constitution body/mind type was:

_____

(Vata-Pitta, Pitta-Vata, Kapha-Pitta, etc.)

What Type Am I?

Once you have scored the questionnaires, look at the numbers and compare them. Scores fall into two basic categories. First, if your highest score in both tests is the same, then you are probably that type. *Example*: a high Pitta score (on both tests) with the next highest number being Kapha would be seen as a Pitta-kapha (big P, little k, Pk). You would then follow the Pitta Program. However, if Test I results (your *present* body/mind type) showed the highest number to be different from Test II (your birth constitution), then you are showing a probable imbalance in the area of the highest score in Test I. *Example*: let's say your Test I score was higher in the Kapha column, next Pitta, then Vata. However, Test II shows your Pitta score as higher, then Kapha, then Vata. This would suggest that you are probably a Pitta-kapha by birth with a Kapha imbalance. In this instance you would need to follow the Kapha program because that is the area of your present imbalance. A Kapha program reduces Kapha while increasing Pitta and Vata simultaneously. You would follow the Kapha program until your weight and other symptoms of imbalance came back into alignment with your birth constitution.

Application of Diagnosis

Once you have figured out which body type you were at birth, you then need to determine what your body type is now and follow the program for that type (the number that is highest in your questionnaire). For example, if you now are a Pitta-kapha (Pk), and in the second questionnaire (birth constitution) you were more Kapha-pitta (Kp), you would follow a Pitta-reducing program to bring your body back into alignment with your birth constitution. In other words, a Vata program is designed to decrease the Vata Effect in the physiology of those following the program. This is because a Vata type will naturally tend to become too Vata; the Pitta program similarly is designed to decrease the Pitta Effect and the Kapha program the Kapha Effect, for the same reason.

My birth constitution Body/Mind Type was:

_____

enter information from page 131

My acquired (present) Body/Mind Type is:

_____

enter information from page 121

Program to Follow:

  _____ Vata Program
  _____ Pitta Program
  _____ Kapha Program

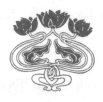

Chapter 14

BODY TYPE ZONE
PROGRAMS FOR HEALTH

Among the several ways to find balance and regain
health, all have as the first requirement our willing participation. What we do for ourselves in our daily practice is
much more important for improving our health than anything a doctor can do. Healthy practices must include proper
daily routine, diet, exercise, and understanding the principles
of wholeness. A doctor's treatment becomes necessary when
we are unable to recover our health through our own efforts.
The value of this treatment is temporary, however, when we
allow ourselves to go out of balance through improper diet,
exercise, daily routine and lack of preventive maintenance.
There is no substitute for right living. In the long run only we
are responsible for our health.

What Will Living in My
Body Type Zone Do for Me?)

The Body Type Zone Programs are designed to:
- Help us understand how and why to nurture our inner
  nature
- Create natural health

- Be complete and wholistic in nature
- Enhance well-being through regularity
- Provide long-term benefits
- Help us take an active part in our own health care

What to Do

At this point you should know which of the seven basic body types you are: Vata pitta (Vp), Vata kapha (Vk), Pitta vata (Pv), Pitta kapha (Pk), Kapha vata (Kv), Kapha pitta (Kp), or VataPittaKapha (VPK). If your resulting high scores from Test I and Test II are the same you would obviously follow the program for that body type. If your test scores in Test I (acquired body/mind type) are different from those of Test II (birth constitution), you would follow the program for the highest score in Test I. As we have said, the Pitta Program will decrease Pitta, for example, and the Kapha Program is designed to reduce Kapha, Vata to reduce Vata, because each constitution tends to increase naturally.

To be sure you are not in denial about your condition, go over your test scores another time. If they show you to be primarily a Pitta (birth constitution - Test II) but you are overweight, your best bet would be the Kapha program to reduce Kapha, not a Pitta program. Making an incorrect dosha diagnosis is the most common cause of failure of the Body Type Zone Program. If we don't diagnose the right dosha we probably cannot determine which of the Body Type Zone Programs we should be following.

Apply each practice in your Body Type Program to your daily life as best you can, one at a time. A week or two is usually required to become comfortable with each practice before adding the next. Vatas, don't rush and read ahead. Pittas, don't try to do it all in one day. Kaphas, don't put it off until next week. As you do each practice, try to understand what effect it will have on your own physiology. Once you realize the effect, decide if it feels good to you. If it does, continue it.

The applications that follow are the ones I have found most effective in my clinical practice, and the most valuable and practical over all.

Body Type Zone Programs

The Body Type Zone Program for each type contains recommendations for daily habits and practices. In my chiropractic practice, I used to give my patients all these recommendations on their first visit. Naively, I expected they would *practice* them. Of course, they were so overwhelmed that they couldn't get going on the program at all. I now tell my patients that this information is like learning to play the guitar: I'll teach the D chord and the G chord this week and if you learn them by next week, I'll teach A7 and B minor (I have a degree in Music Education). If you know anything about music, you know that many pieces can be played with just these chords. But if you don't learn the first two chords, the next chords won't matter much. As when learning to play an instrument, you will need to practice the practices until they become second nature, a part of your day. When you can do this, you will be nurturing your inner nature – the real YOU.

Each Body Type Zone Program is broken down into four parts. It is suggested you practice Part I for a week or two until you feel comfortable, then move on to Part II, Part III, etc., applying each set of practices for a week or more before moving on to the next. At the end of four or so weeks, you will be routinely practicing the full Body Type Zone Program for your body type.

To find your balance and regain your health, the first requirement is your willing participation. What we do for ourselves in our daily practice is much more important to our overall health than anything a doctor can do. Our healthy practices must include proper daily routine, diet, exercise and the understanding of the principles of wholeness. A doctor's treatment becomes necessary when we are unable to recover our health through our own efforts; however, even a doctor's treatment is temporary when we allow ourselves to go out of balance through improper diet, exercise, daily routine and lack of preventive care. There is no substitute for right living. In the end, only we are responsible for our health.

Practices for Balancing Vata

Vata Effect tends toward a faster metabolic rate and catabolism (tissue reducing and constricting). The following practices reduce the Vata Effect by increasing the Pitta Effect and Kapha Effect. These practices calm the nervous system. Remember, Vatas need to *relax*; meditation is great for Vatas!

Part I: Regular Routines

• Regular Routine: No matter what body type we are, to balance an out-of-balance Vata we must establish a regular routine. Most people are not accustomed to having a regular routine and few know why it is important. Because this Vata part of our nature is so sensitive and changeable, we can find ourselves stressed by our daily hectic lives, leading to symptoms of anxiety, nervousness, and restlessness – a Vata Effect. The sympathetic nervous system, once stimulated, needs to be reset. Vata sets the rhythm to which the rest of the body dances; therefore, if we are over-stimulated we need to slow the music. We can do this by having a regular schedule of activities. It is best to get up and go to bed at about the same time every day. As well, we need to be especially regular about each aspect of our diet, rest, and bowel habits. Each of these should occur at about the same time each day. When we eat our meals at the same time every day, our digestion stays strong and regular. This helps to regulate the insulin/glucagon balance and the agni (digestive fire). Exercise should be consistent and practiced at the same time each day as well. Our inner nature will appreciate this subtle yet powerful practice of regularity. This does not mean we become rigid, it means we become more flexible. Regularity is the oil that lubricates the dry wheel of Vata. Balancing Vata also helps bring the Pitta and Kapha part of our natures back into alignment, as Vata is movement and all changes involve a Vata component.

Therefore, to balance Vata, emphasize a *regular routine*. For the practice of good health, regularity is of the utmost importance to a Vata.

• Write it Down: Begin by jotting down a schedule to follow for the first few weeks. After awhile, it will become an easy, healthy habit.

• Hot Water Routine: For general purification, drinking hot water frequently throughout the day is beneficial to decrease the cold quality of Vata. Heat the water and carry it in a thermos while at work or on the go and drink a sip or two every half hour. This program does not work if you drink three or four cups in the morning and no more until night. Drink a little over a long period for the results to be effective.

• Fennel After Meals: chewing fennel seeds (about 1/4 tsp.) after lunch and dinner will aid the digestive process. Chew them thoroughly, keeping them in your mouth for some time, then swallow.

• Staying Warm: the nature of Vata is cold. Vatas need to keep themselves warm and toasty and avoid being chilled. Though this may seem a bit simplistic, a Vata type just can't afford to get cold. Even drinking cold drinks can chill the body and decrease its ability to create a strong digestive fire.

Part II: Vata-Reducing Diet

We must give extra attention to establishing a balanced, wholesome diet that will include fresh, good-quality, delicious and nutritious foods. In Ayurvedic practice, food is freshly prepared just before eating. Of course, fast foods or packaged foods, preservatives, leftovers, or foods of little nutritional value are not part of this practice. In our present culture, however, avoiding these foods without conscious effort is difficult. By looking at the qualities of Vata, Pitta and Kapha and the effect a food has on our system, we can decide what foods are good for our body type.

Vata has a natural tendency to increase. When it becomes out of balance, we need to decrease the Vata in our system. The Vata-reducing diet will decrease the tendency of Vata to accumulate. We want to reduce the Vata qualities of cold, dry, light, quick, rough, irregular. The recommended Vata diet includes foods that are warm and moist to counteract the cold and dry qualities of Vata. This section contains a list of suggested foods.

- Increase foods that are warm, heavier, oilier, as they increase the Pitta and Kapha Effect.
- Reduce foods that are cold, dry, lighter as they increase the Vata Effect, which we are trying to reduce.
- Increase foods that are sweet, sour, salty as they increase the Pitta and Kapha Effect.
- Reduce foods that are spicy, bitter, and astringent as they increase the Vata Effect.
- You may eat larger quantities of food, but of course not more than you can easily digest. Eat on a regular basis. Vatas often forget to eat (Pittas find this hard to believe). Remember, Vata's digestive system is more irregular in nature, so what you can eat one day may not be easily digested the next.
- Dairy products (in small quantities) decrease the Vata Effect and are therefore permissible.
- All sweeteners (in small quantities) decrease the Vata Effect, and are therefore permissible.
- Oils reduce the Vata Effect and are used successfully by the Vata type.
- Grains: rice and wheat are good for Vata, but reduce barley, corn, millet, buckwheat, rye, and oats.
- Fruits: favor sweet, sour, or heavy fruits such as bananas, avocados, grapes, oranges, cherries, peaches, mangoes, papayas, melons, berries, plums, and pineapples. Reduce dry or light fruits (apples, pears, dried fruits).
- Use cooked vegetables rather than raw, as they are eas-

ier for Vata to digest. Occasionally Vata may have salad or raw foods, but in general, cooked foods will be easier to digest.

- Spices that help reduce Vata are cinnamon, black pepper, ginger, cardamom, cumin, salt, cloves, and mustard seed.

- Nuts can be good for Vata if chewed well enough to be digested.

- Avoid or reduce beans (except tofu) as they are harder for Vatas to digest. The Vata has more difficulty digesting protein than Pitta or Kapha, which results in undigested food mass, gas, and bloating – the Vata Effect.

- Vata still needs an adequate supply of protein. Meat, fish, chicken, turkey and seafood may be fine in small amounts if chewed well.

- Eating meals in a settled and relaxed environment is important for all body types, but especially so for the Vata. Watching TV, reading, or driving in a car while eating takes our mind and our body off the task at hand. As well, we don't enjoy the food as much because we are enjoying something else or are entirely distracted. It is also good to relax after a meal before resuming activity, allowing the body to focus on the first stages of digestion. These practices are important for improving digestion and allowing the body to heal.

- Vegetarian diet: according to Ayurveda, a diet that is low or lower in meat (heavy protein) is a healthier diet. This is because meat, if not digested, creates ama, or undigested food mass, which the body must deal with in some manner as accumulation of ama results in symptoms of disease. For the Vata type eating meat can be a problem anyway. Because Vata has difficulty digesting food in general and protein in specific, many Vata types have quite naturally become vegetarians. It is recommended that meat eaters cut down on consumption. This can be done gradually, over time. After awhile you can decide whether to continue to eat meat at all, or occasionally and in small amounts. Many people switch to eating fish and poultry as their main menu item. However, if you eat as much chicken and fish as you ate meat, you are really not improving your diet or health.

- It is best that Vata types eliminate caffeine from the diet altogether. Caffeine is like rocket fuel to a Vata and it will shoot them far into space. Caffeine stimulates the sympathetic nervous system and activates the adrenal glands. A Vata is already halfway there (out in space). Drinking caffeine can only aggravate the Vata condition. A Kapha can handle it better, but still it is not the best.

- Including Ghee in Diet: include ghee (clarified butter) in your daily diet. It can be used on bread, grains, vegetables, etc. Ghee is available in many natural food stores, and is easily prepared at home. *Note: individuals who have a known or suspected problem with high lipids, (high cholesterol) should restrict ghee in their diet.*

- Ginger in the Diet: ginger can be used quite successfully by most body types if used properly. Ginger is a warming spice, so it is very good for the Vata type. Fresh ginger is best. It can be used in daily cooking in a variety of recipes, or peeled, sliced, and simmered in filtered water to make a warming, healing ginger tea.

- Remember, for the Vata / Metabolic Type I Zone, the ratio of proteins to carbohydrates to fats should be 20/40/40:

20 % protein

40% carbohydrate

40% fat

Part III: Nurturing

- Warm Water in the Morning: to stimulate elimination in the morning, start the day with a glass of warm water. This practice stimulates peristalsis – the muscle contractions in the colon that begin emptying the bowel. Be very regular with this practice. The Vata physiology is more prone to constipation than Pitta or Kapha, and extra consideration must be given to proper elimination.

- Quietness: the irregularity of a Vata's nature is diminished and soothed through quiet relaxation, contemplation, and meditation. These practices help calm the frazzled sympathetic nerves of the over-stimulated Vata. The regular practice of quiet relaxation will decrease the sympathetic nervous stimulation and increase the parasympathetic nervous system response to allow the body to nourish itself and heal.

- Lunch as Main Meal: in this country, this practice is difficult simply because most of us are at work at mid-day and must either bring our lunch or grab a quick meal at a restaurant. However, we should eat the heaviest meal in the middle of the day as our digestive fire is highest between 11:00 a.m. and 2:00 p.m. Night-time digestive cycles are more for the later stages of digestion, not the early stages. All of us have experienced eating late and getting up the next morning feeling full and bloated. The food has not been well digested and still remains to be processed. This causes a subtle but potentially powerful disruption of the body's ability to process food, leading to all sorts of symptoms that are seemingly unrelated to when and how much we eat. The evening meal, then, should be lighter, with at least two hours between eating and going to bed.

- Rest: these days, many things will excite us and spur us on to movement; but remember, if we rest frequently, our body can recover more quickly and we will be able to do more with greater strength and stamina after rest. Vata types just keep going until they collapse. If they rested a couple of times a day, they would increase their clarity and decrease anxiety.

- Exercise: exercise is good for the Vata but should not be overdone. Mild yoga postures and tai chi are perfect. Avoid the wind and cold outdoors; you need to stay warm. Bundle up when appropriate. Vata does very well with mild daily exercise that does not lead to labored breathing, excessive perspiration, or fatigue. Walking is good, riding a bike is great, swimming can be wonderful – but all of these should be done with low intensity and for shorter distances than we might expect. You should feel enlivened at the end of your exercise, not wrung out.

- Daily Sesame Oil Massage: before going to bed each night, apply warm sesame oil to your body. You can oil your entire body or just your feet, hands, and abdomen as time permits. This practice is very soothing to a Vata's physiology. Follow the self-massage with a warm bath and you will find yourself sleeping like a baby. This is very powerful in reducing the Vata Effect.

- Early to Bed: is hard for a Vata. They get wound up and just keep going. Because they do not allow themselves the wind-down time before sleep, they are not able to go to bed at a decent hour (that hour, by the way is about 10:00 p.m.). If we go to bed by ten, we can wake up by five or six, far more refreshed. This is important for all types, but especially so for Vata. The Vata nervous system heals itself when it gets enough rest and sleep. Because the Vata has a tendency toward such frazzled nerves, getting a good night's rest is very important.

Part IV: Exercises for Health and Well-Being

- Meditation: the practice of daily meditation can help bring contentment and peace into your life. It is detoxification for the mind. Because there are so many methods of meditation, it may be helpful to take a lesson or two.

- No Anger, No Worry: for many of us, this seems impossible; but, as much as possible, we need to avoid situations that tend to cause worry and upset. If our job creates anger and upset, we may need to find a different job. If we are constantly worried about finances, we may need to reduce our overhead to reduce stress. If we are angry with someone, we need to forgive them. Anger, upset, and worry create an imbalance in the body and will aggravate any condition.

- Forgiveness: the physiology of forgiveness is more powerful than any medicine. There is nothing we can do that will help more than to forgive those with whom we are angry, even though we believe they may deserve punishment! The physiology of resentment creates illness wherever it goes. Healing means forgiveness: forgiveness means healing. Forgiveness reduces the Vata and Pitta Effect; Kapha seems to have a greater capacity for forgiveness. Forgiveness is not always easy, but it's necessary for well-being.

- Avoid Late Night Activities: when we begin a project in the early evening we engage our mind and emotions with the intensity to follow through to completion whatever we are doing. This increases the Vata and Pitta Effect on our physiology and will tend to keep us from falling asleep. When we do fall asleep, we will often have a restless night. The early evening should be the winding down part of the day as we decrease our more intense activities.

- The Practice of Yoga: Yoga postures (asanas) are specially good for the Vata type. These exercises will help restore mind/body coordination, and are generally appropriate for all three body types. See Resource Guide for books on Yoga.

- Sun Salutations: the Yoga postures called Sun Salutations are an excellent way to start the day. If done gently, without strain, most people can benefit from these postures, adding flexibility and strength to the whole body. Start with up to six sets of sun salutations. Remember, Vata, don't exercise to the point of fatigue or heavy breathing. This will aggravate the Vata condition rather than help it.

- Rest During Menstrual Cycle (Female): According to Ayurveda, resting during the first day or two of her menstrual cycle is important for a woman. If total rest is not possible, getting as much rest as possible during these days is a must. This may be difficult in our present culture. Most employers do not look favorably on our missing work to stay home and rest. Do what you can; rest when you can.

Balancing the Pitta Effect

All of the following reduce the Pitta Effect by increasing the Vata Effect and/or Kapha Effect. These practices generally have a cooling effect on the digestive system. Remember, Pittas need to chill out and moderate. Pitta Effect tends toward fast and strong metabolism with emphasis on transformation (tissue changing).

Part I: Regular Routines

- Regular Routine: even Pitta will benefit from regular routine. Because the Vata part of our nature is so sensitive and changeable, we can find ourselves stressed out by our daily hectic lives, leading to symptoms of anxiety, nervousness, and restlessness, a Vata Effect. Yes, this can happen to a Pitta. The sympathetic nervous system, once stimulated, needs to be reset. Vata sets the rhythm to which the rest of the body dances; therefore, if we are over-stimulated we need to slow the song. We can do this with a regular schedule of activities. Pittas, as well as Vatas, benefit from going to bed and getting up at the same time every day. Being especially regular about each aspect of diet, rest, and bowel habits is also important. When we eat our meals at the same time every day our digestion stays strong and regular. This helps to regulate the agni (digestive fire) and the insulin/glucagon balance. Exercise should be consistent and practiced at the same time each day. Our inner nature will appreciate this subtle yet powerful practice of regularity. Balancing our Vata tendencies also helps bring the Pitta and Kapha part of our natures back into alignment. Each body type must take care not to increase the Vata Effect too much.

To reinforce a daily routine, begin by **writing down a schedule** to follow for the first few weeks. After awhile, it will become a healthy habit.

• Hot Water Routine: as a Pitta, increasing heat is generally not the prescribed course of action – unless we are experiencing ama, or an increased toxic load. In the colder months, drinking a sip or two of hot water every half hour may help to gently detoxify the system. You may heat the water in a coffee pot and carry it in a thermos while at work or on the go. Don't, however, get overheated. Pitta should use this hot-water regimen only while working to detox the body.

• Fennel after Meals: as for Vata, chewing fennel seeds (about 1/4 tsp.) after lunch and dinner aids the digestive process for all body types. Chew them thoroughly, keeping them in your mouth for some time, then swallow.

• Staying Cool: as we have said, the nature of Pitta is hot. Pitta needs to stay cool and calm and avoid being overheated in temperature or in emotions. Though this may seem a bit simplistic, a Pitta type just cannot afford to get any hotter.

• Practice of Moderation: the key to balancing Pitta is finding moderation. A Pitta imbalance is likely to occur when we have pushed ourselves beyond our limits, beyond our capacity to recover. The fiery inner nature of a Pitta is driving and competitively aggressive. Fire can warm us or it can consume us. Balancing the fire energy is about going fast enough and far enough to get the job done without burning up on re-entry; it is about realizing the need to balance extreme workaholic tendencies while taking the time to stop and see what we have produced, to admire it, to nurture it. Vatas and Pittas both can get burned out from overdoing it – so cool down.

• Cooling Down: a cool compress to the forehead and/or back of the neck can benefit an over- heated Pitta. Drinking plenty of liquid in warm weather is also helpful.

Part II: Pitta-Reducing Diet

The Pitta diet would include foods that are cooler to counteract the hot qualities of Pitta. A list of suggested foods will follow in the next section. Extra attention must be given to establishing a balanced yet wholesome diet that includes foods that are fresh, of good quality, delicious and nutritious. The food should be freshly prepared at each meal. Fast foods or packaged foods, preservatives, leftovers, or foods of little nutritional value are not part of an Ayurvedic dietary practice. In our present culture however, avoiding these foods without conscious effort is difficult.

Pittas need to decrease the amount of Pitta in the system when it is overflowing the cup. Foods listed below will decrease the natural tendency of Pitta to accumulate. Stick to the Pitta diet recommendations as much as possible. Begin to understand that the food we eat directly affects our health. Note that a Pitta diet is one that reduces the Pitta Effect (hot, sharp, moist, moving, fluid) yet increases the Vata and Kapha Effect. By looking at the qualities of Vata, Pitta and Kapha and observing the effect a food has on our system, we can determine what foods are good for our body type.

- Increase foods that are cooler, lighter, and less oily, as they increase the Vata and Kapha Effect.
- Reduce foods that are hotter and oilier as they increase the Pitta Effect.
- Increase foods that are sweet, bitter, or astringent as they increase the Vata and Kapha Effect.

- Reduce foods that are pungent, sour, or salty as they increase the Pitta Effect.

- Do not overeat. Pitta has a strong appetite (which can be excessive) and can overload the digestive system with too much volume. Like Vatas, Pittas must also eat on a regular basis.

- Moderate dairy, milk, butter and ghee are acceptable for Pitta, though they may increase the Pitta Effect. Dairy is high fat; therefore, the tendency of Pittas to have difficulty with fat metabolism will tend to increase. Moderation is key.

- All sweeteners, except honey and molasses, decrease the Pitta Effect.

- Avoid yogurt, cheese, sour cream as they increase the Pitta Effect.

- Reduce oils generally as they increase the Pitta Effect, especially sesame, almond, and corn oil. Oils more favorable to Pitta are olive, sunflower, and coconut.

- Wheat, rice, barley, and oats are good as they decrease the Pitta Effect. Reduce corn, millet and rye.

- Favor sweet fruits such as grapes, cherries, melons, avocado, coconut, pomegranates, mangoes, oranges, pineapples, and plums as they reduce the Pitta Effect. Reduce sour fruits such as grapefruits, olives, and papayas as they increase the Pitta Effect.

- Occasional salads and raw vegetables are fine, but in general, cooked foods are easier for the Pitta system to digest.

- Reduce nuts in your diet, especially cashews and peanuts, as they are heavy in oils, which increase the Pitta Effect.

- Reduce beans, as they are hard for the Pitta type to digest. Acceptable beans are chickpeas, mung beans, soybean, and kidney.

- Favor vegetables such as broccoli, cauliflower, asparagus, cucumber, green leafy vegetables, green beans, zucchini, pumpkins, celery, okra, lettuce, potatoes, and sweet potatoes. Avoid hot peppers, tomatoes, onions, garlic, radishes, spinach, carrots, and beets, as they tend to increase the Pitta Effect.

- Acceptable spices are cardamom, fennel, cinnamon, coriander, black pepper (in small quantities). Reduce cumin, cloves, celery seed, ginger, salt, fenugreek and mustard seed as they tend to increase the Pitta Effect.

- Avoid chili peppers and cayenne pepper as they dramatically increase the Pitta Effect.

- In general, reduce hot things in your diet.

- Poultry (chicken, pheasant, and turkey) is preferable for Pitta, though they can be vegetarians with little trouble.

- Reduce beef, seafood, and eggs as they increase the Pitta Effect.

- Including Ghee in Diet: Pittas may include moderate amounts of ghee (clarified butter) in the daily diet. It can be used sparingly on bread, grains, or vegetables in place of margarine or butter. Ghee is easy to prepare at home, though it is also available in many natural food stores. *Note: individuals who have a known or suspected problem with fat metabolism, high cholesterol, or high triglycerides should restrict ghee in their diet.*

- Vegetarian Diet: according to Ayurveda, a diet that is low or lower in meat (heavy protein) is a healthier diet for all body types. This is because meat, if not properly digested, creates undigested food mass (ama) which the body must deal with in some manner, as the accumulation of ama results in symptoms of disease. Pitta may not experience the same difficulty in digesting meat as Vata, unless a digestive disturbance is already present. Pittas, if imbalanced, may have more difficulty with meat because of the fat. Though meat is high in protein it also may have a large fat content; therefore, it makes sense to cut down on meat consumption. This can be done gradually, over time, and after awhile you may decide to eat meat only occasionally and in smaller amounts or forego meat altogether. Many people switch to fish and poultry as their main menu items. If they eat chicken and fish as much as they ate meat, however, they are not greatly improving their diet or health.

- Eat in a relaxed setting: eating meals in a settled and relaxed environment is important for all body types. As with Vata, watching TV, reading, or driving a car while eating takes our mind and our body off the task at hand. As well, we don't enjoy the food as much because we are distracted or enjoying something else. A Pitta type is more likely doing something that requires competition, not good for digestion. It is also important to relax after a meal before resuming activity, allowing the body to focus on the first stages of digestion. These practices are important for improving digestion and allowing the body to heal.

- Remember, for the Pitta / Metabolic Type II Zone, the ratio of proteins to carbohydrates to fats should be 30/50/20:

  30 % protein

  50 % carbohydrate

  20% fat

Part III: Nurturing the Self

- No Stimulants: giving a stimulant to a Pitta is like pouring gasoline on a fire. A Pitta who drinks caffeine may drive his already hot, aggressive nature to a boiling point. If you show signs of a Pitta imbalance, including anger and irritation, consider decreasing the stimulating substances in your life such as coffee, chocolate, tea, and tobacco. Everyone else in your life will appreciate this as well.

- Warm Water in the Morning: the Pitta physiology has

an increase of bile production that stimulates regular peristalsis (the muscle contractions in the colon that begin the emptying process of the bowel). However, even Pittas sometimes exhibit the Vata tendency toward constipation. If so, you may stimulate your elimination in the morning by starting the day with a glass of warm water.

- Quietness: Pittas have as part of their nature a Vata component which can be soothed by quiet relaxation, contemplation and meditation. The practice of quietness helps calm the frazzled sympathetic nerves of the over-stimulated Pitta-vata. A regular practice of quiet relaxation will decrease the sympathetic nervous stimulation and increase the parasympathetic nervous system response to allow the body to nourish itself and heal. For the Pitta, moderation of aggressive tendencies is essential. Quietly allowing for things to happen in life will increase their mental and emotional health.

- Lunch as Main Meal: in this country taking our main meal at mid-day is often difficult because most of us are at work and must either bring lunch or eat quickly at a restaurant. However, because our digestive fire is highest between 11:00 a.m. and 2:00 p.m., it makes sense to eat our heaviest meal in the middle of the day. All of us have experienced eating late and getting up the next morning feeling full and bloated, meaning that our food was not well-digested. This causes a subtle but potentially powerful disruption of our body's ability to process food, which can lead to symptoms seemingly unrelated to when and how much we eat. Unlike Vata, a Pitta is usually very hungry at mealtime. Even after eating a large midday meal a Pitta will want a full evening meal. However, the evening meal should always be light with at least two hours between eating and going to bed.

- Rest: frequent rest enables the body to recover more quickly and allows us to do more, with greater strength and stamina, after resting. As with Vata, Pittas will typically continue on well past their ability to recover well. If they rest a couple of times a day they will experience increased clarity and decreased fatigue.

- Exercise: Pitta needs more vigorous exercise than a Vata. A Pitta can enjoy working out on a regular basis, in the outdoors, in all kinds of weather, but should not get overheated. Exertion should be moderate. We should feel enlivened after exercise not wrung out. Pittas need to exercise but should not overdo it. Walking is very beneficial to all three body types; riding a bike and swimming are also great, and all can be done with a good level of intensity. Regular aerobic exercise and/or weight training are good for Pitta, and moderate to heavy physical labor can also be good if not overdone. The fiery quality of Pitta may cause us to do too much, to compete with ourselves beyond rest and reason. Pittas need to move and stay fit, but overdoing it will only weaken them.

- Daily Oil Massage: before going to bed each night, apply slightly warmed coconut oil to your body. You can do your entire body or just your feet, hands, and abdomen as time permits. This is very soothing to the Vata part of your physiology. Follow the self-massage by a warm bath and you will find yourself sleeping like a baby. This practice, using cooling coconut oil, helps to moderate the Pitta Effect.

- Winding Down: Pittas need a period of rest and relaxation at the end of the day to balance their natural "on the go" tendency. While a Vata's tendency to be on the move is perhaps less purposeful (cleaning an already clean area, for instance), a Pitta's is more aggressive (they may decide to take over their town). An irritated Pitta needs to wind down slowly and come to a comfortable place of rest, relaxation, and calm. Just as for the Vata type, meditation can be most helpful.

- Early to Bed: is as hard for a Pitta as a Vata. They both

get wound up and just keep going. Because they do not allow themselves the wind-down time before sleep, they are often unable to go to bed at a reasonable hour (about 10:00 p.m.). The nervous system heals itself when we rest and sleep; our digestion completes its processing during sleep as well. If we go to bed by ten we can awaken by five or six far more refreshed. This is important for Pitta and all body types.

Part IV: Exercises for Health and Well-Being

- Meditation: for a Pitta, daily meditation can help bring contentment and peace to life. It is detoxification for the mind. Because meditation comes in many forms, it may be helpful to take a lesson or two to find the method most suitable for you.

- No Anger, No Worry: this is difficult for many people. For a Pitta, anger is second nature. If our job creates anger and upset, we may need to find a different job. If we are upset about finances, we may need to reduce overhead to reduce the stress. Pittas especially will want to avoid situations that tend to cause anger and upset. Rather than carrying anger in our body, we need to forgive and (try to) forget.

- Forgiveness: the physiology of forgiveness is more powerful than any existing medicine. Letting go of anger and resentment (the Pitta Effect) is very healing. *Forgiveness* is very healing – it actually reduces the Pitta Effect. Forgiveness is not easy, but it's necessary. Kapha has the greatest capacity for forgiveness, but all can do it.

- Avoid Late Night Activities: as with Vata, when a Pitta begins a project in the early evening, the mind and emotions are engaged. A Pitta does not like to go to bed without having accomplished something so will likely stay up until the project is complete. This stimulation will make sleep difficult. The early evening should be the winding-down part of the day; this is a time to decrease more intense activities, not to begin them.

- Sun Salutations: as with Vata, a Yoga exercise called Sun Salutations is an excellent way to start the day. If done gently, without strain, these postures can be done by most people and will add flexibility and strength to the entire body. Start with up to six sets of sun salutations. Remember, Pitta, don't overdo.

- Rest During Menstrual Cycle (Female): Pitta women may have a heavier flow than Vata, so taking care to rest during the first couple of days of the menstrual cycle is very important. If total rest is not possible, getting as much rest as possible during these days is a must. However, if you are working, your employer may not think it a good idea to stay home during this time, and you may not feel able to take days off and forfeit the income. However, do what you can; rest when you can.

Practices for Balancing Kapha

Kapha tends toward slower and more sluggish metabolism with emphasis on anabolism (tissue building). The following recommendations reduce the Kapha Effect by increasing the Vata Effect and/or Pitta Effect. These practices generally have a warming and stimulating effect on the digestive system. Remember that Kaphas need stimulation and warmth to offset their sluggish system.

Part I: Regular Routines

• Regular Routine: even if we are a Kapha body type, to balance our Vata tendencies (which we all have) a regular routine is recommended. Balancing our Vata tendencies also helps bring the Pitta and Kapha parts of our nature into alignment. A Kapha type needs to practice regular routines while simultaneously nurturing the Kapha nature. Because the Vata part of our nature is so sensitive and changeable we can find ourselves stressed out by our daily hectic lives, leading to symptoms of anxiety, nervousness, and restlessness, a Vata Effect – which even a Kapha can experience. Though

Kapha is less prone to over-stimulation, we may still need to slow down the song. We can do this by maintaining a regular schedule of activities. It is best to get up and go to bed at the same time every day and be especially regular about diet, rest, and bowel habits. Each of these should occur at about the same time each day. When we eat our meals at the same time every day our digestion stays strong and regular, helping to regulate the digestive fire and the insulin/glucagon balance. Exercise (yes, Kapha, you need to exercise) should be consistent and at the same time each day as well. To help the practice of regular routines, begin by writing down a schedule for the first few weeks. After awhile, these routines will become a healthy habit. Your inner nature will appreciate this subtle yet powerful practice of regularity.

• Hot Water Routine: for general purification and to decrease the cold quality of Kapha, drinking hot water frequently throughout the day is beneficial. As a Kapha, increasing heat helps decrease a toxic build-up in the body. Heat the water in a coffee pot and carry it in a thermos while at work or on the go, and drink a sip or two or more every half hour. The program does not work if you drink three or four cups in the morning and none until night. Drink a little over a long period for the results to be effective.

• Fennel after meals: chewing fennel seeds (about 1/4 tsp.) after lunch and dinner will aid the digestive process. Chew them thoroughly, keeping them in your mouth for some time, then swallow.

• Staying Warm: the nature of Kapha is cold. Kaphas need to keep themselves warm and toasty and avoid being chilled. Though this may seem a bit simplistic, a Kapha type just can't afford to get any cooler. They are already moving slow enough as it is.

Part II: Kapha-Reducing Diet

A Kapha diet is one that reduces the Kapha Effect (heavy, cold, dull, moist, stable, sticky) yet increases the Vata and Pitta Effect. By looking at the qualities of Vata, Pitta and

Kapha (Chapter 3) and the effect of foods on our system, we can determine what foods are good for our body type. Perhaps we can then begin to understand that the nature of food directly affects our health.

Kapha can take a diet of liquids or liquefied foods as often as they like. They may choose a liquid diet as frequently as once a week or once a month. A liquid diet reduces stress on the digestive system and helps promote better assimilation. Women may choose a liquid diet on the first day of menstruation. This is not a fast; we may include anything we like in the diet as long as it is first liquefied. Because a liquid diet is generally used for purification, using foods that are fresh and wholesome is best. Common items to include are soups, freshly made fruit juices or fresh vegetable juices prepared from carrots or beets, herbal teas, or hot water with lemon; however, you are not limited to these items.

The Kapha diet includes warmer foods to counteract the cold qualities of Kapha. Extra attention must be given to establishing a balanced, yet wholesome, diet that includes foods that are fresh, of good quality, delicious and nutritious. In Ayurveda, this means that the food should be freshly prepared right before eating. And of course fast foods or packaged foods, preservatives, leftovers, or foods of little nutritional value are not part of the Ayurvedic practice. As we have said, this may be difficult in our present culture, and may require conscious effort.

Foods on the following list will decrease the tendency of Kapha to accumulate. Try to stick to this diet as much as possible. This is a diet designed to nourish and detoxify at the same time. A Kapha-reducing diet is light and favors steamed vegetables, beans, hot spices with light grains that produce an increased Vata and Pitta Effect and is more diuretic (water-releasing) in nature. For Kaphas fasting or eating liquid foods may be appropriate for a day or two to give the digestive tract a rest.

- Increase foods that are warmer, lighter, and less oily as they increase the Vata and Pitta Effect.

- Reduce foods that are colder and heavier as they increase the Kapha Effect, which we do not want to do if we already have too much Kapha.

- Increase foods that are pungent, bitter, and astringent as they increase the Vata and Pitta Effect.

- Reduce foods that are sweet, sour, or salty as they increase the Kapha Effect.

- Do not overeat. Kapha has a less intense appetite than Pitta, but certainly can overeat. Most people think that Kapha, the heaviest of the body types, would have the biggest appetite; however, Pittas win in that category. Kaphas are larger and heavier because their digestive system is very efficient. A Vata can eat more than a Kapha and put on no weight. A Kapha just looks at food and there goes another belt notch. Kaphas inherently know that there are differences in metabolism. It all relates to the preponderance of endodermal tissue (which becomes the lining of the gastrointestinal system) and their hormone response to carbohydrates. Though Vatas and Pittas must eat regularly, a Kapha can afford to skip a meal, maybe even two.

- Dairy products (milk, butter and ghee) are not good for the Kapha physiology because they increase the Kapha Effect. Dairy is high in fat and milk sugar (lactose), therefore increasing the tendency of Kaphas to have difficulty with fat and sugar metabolism. Minimal dairy is recommended.

- All sweeteners, except honey, should be reduced as they increase the Kapha Effect.

- Reduce oils generally as they increase the Kapha Effect.

- Grains: barley, millet, buckwheat, and rye are good for Kapha. Sweet grains such as rice, wheat, corn and oats should be avoided.

- Fruits: reduce heavy or sour fruits such as bananas, coconuts, pineapples, figs, dates, avocados, oranges, and melons.

- Salads, raw vegetables, and cooked vegetables decrease the Kapha Effect.
- Vegetables are generally good, although reducing sweet potatoes, tomatoes, cucumbers, and zucchini is best.
- Reduce nuts as they are heavy in oils that increase the Kapha Effect.
- Beans are usually good, except soy and kidney which should be reduced.
- Increase pungent spices (hot spices) such as cumin, cloves, ginger, and mustard seed as they tend to increase the Pitta Effect and reduce the Kapha Effect.
- Meat and fish: reduce red meat and pork as well as fish and seafood in general.
- Eat in a relaxed setting: eating meals in a settled and relaxed environment is important for all body types, even a Kapha. Watching TV, reading, or driving in a car while eating takes your mind and your body off the task at hand. A Kapha type is more likely to be sitting in front of the television eating dinner, which detracts from the taste of the food – something a Kapha really enjoys. It is also good to relax after a meal before resuming activity, allowing the body to focus on the first stages of digestion. These practices are important for improving digestion and allowing the body to heal.
- Vegetarian Diet: as we have noted, a diet low or lower in meat (heavy protein) is a healthier diet. This is because meat, if not digested, creates ama, or undigested food mass, which the body must deal with in some manner. Accumulation of ama results in symptoms of disease. For the Kapha type, eating meat can be detrimental, as their digestion, though efficient, is slow and sluggish. Though meat is high in protein it also may contain a large amount of fat. In a Kapha's slow digestive system the fat is more efficiently absorbed, leading to weight gain—not good for the imbalanced Kapha. Therefore, as with Vata and Pitta, it is best for Kapha to

cut down on meat consumption. This can be done gradually, over time. After awhile you may decide to eat meat only occasionally and in smaller amounts, or not at all. Switching to fish or poultry as your main menu item may not improve your diet or health if you eat as much chicken and fish as you ate meat.

- Including Ghee in Diet: although Kaphas may include ghee (clarified butter) in their diet, it must be used *sparingly*. Ghee may be prepared at home though it is also available in many natural food stores. *Note: individuals who have a known or suspected problem with fat metabolism, high cholesterol, or high triglycerides should restrict ghee in their diet.*

- Remember, for the Kapha / Metabolic Type III Zone, the ratio of proteins to carbohydrates to fats should be 30/40/30:

  30% protein

  40% carbohydrate

  30% fat

Part III: Nurturing the Self

- Stimulants: giving a stimulant to a Kapha will not increase an energy imbalance as it does in a Vata or Pitta. Though coffee, tea, or other stimulants are not good for us, their effect on the Kapha's system is less damaging. Kaphas can occasionally indulge in caffeine. When they do, it seems to get them off the couch. On a regular basis, however, stimulants are not desirable for our physiology.

- Warm Water in the Morning: to stimulate elimination in the morning, start the day with a glass of warm water. This practice stimulates peristalsis, the muscle contractions in the colon that begin the bowel's emptying process. Be very regular with this practice, as the Kapha physiology is more prone to slow and sluggish digestion and elimination.

- Quietness: Kaphas have a Vata component as part of their nature. The practice of quietness helps calm the frazzled sympathetic nerves that create anxiety and anxiousness (a Vata Effect). The regular practice of quiet relaxation will increase the parasympathetic nervous system and allow the body to nourish itself and replenish. Even Kaphas need this. Quietly allowing for things to happen in life will increase mental and emotional health.

- Lunch as Main Meal: in this country taking our main meal at mid-day is often difficult, because most of us are at work and must either bring lunch or eat quickly at a restaurant. However, because our digestive fire is highest between 11:00 a.m. and 2:00 p.m., it makes sense to eat our heaviest meal in the middle of the day. All of us have experienced eating late in the day and getting up the next morning feeling full and bloated, meaning that our food was not well-digested. This causes a subtle but potentially powerful disruption of our body's ability to process food, which can lead to symptoms seemingly unrelated to when and how much we eat. The evening meal, then, should be light. For a Kapha it should be very light. Allow at least two hours between eating and going to bed.

- Stimulation: Although quietness is necessary to nourish and replenish the body, the key to balancing Kapha is finding things in life that stimulate them. A Kapha imbalance is likely to occur when we have not pushed ourselves up off the couch to experience life. Kapha energy is very earthy, very stable. The inner nature of a Kapha is calm and peaceful. Peaceful is good, stagnant is not. It must have been a Kapha who invented the remote control for the television. To balance the sluggish energy of Kapha we need to wake up the Pitta and Vata part of our nature. We can then get up and go and experience life. Once up and going, the Kapha can go longer and accomplish more than either Vata or Pitta.

- Rest: a Kapha generally knows how to rest. Though Vata types just continue moving until they collapse and Pittas will also go on long past their ability to recover well, a Kapha type knows the beauty of a little rest. For a Kapha, resting a couple of times a day will increase clarity and decrease fatigue and sluggishness.

- Exercise: exercise for the Kapha is not only good, but essential. Exercise is very good for the Kapha's sluggish system. The key is to find an exercise you like. Once found, do it – and do it often. Get into your aerobic zone. It is very stimulating.

- Sesame Oil Massage: before going to bed, you may apply a light, warm, sesame oil to your body. You can massage your entire body or just your feet, hands, and abdomen as time permits. Kaphas do not necessarily need the oil, but can benefit from the deep relaxing benefit of increased restful sleep. Follow the self mas-sage by a warm bath and you will find yourself sleeping like a baby.

- Winding Down: even though the slower, calmer nature of Kapha is almost 'wound down' anyway, they still need to take time to relax before going to bed. While a Vata's tendency is to be on the move and a Pitta's move-ment may have more purpose, Kaphas simply feel that since they are up and running they may as well contin-ue running, since it doesn't happen that often. So they can use a slowing down at the end of the day just as Vata and Pitta.

- Early to Bed: is difficult for a Kapha if they have gotten into the habit of overstimulating late at night. Kaphas can get wound up and just keep going, so they also need to allow themselves a wind-down time before sleep. The best time for that is about 10:00 p.m. If we go to bed by ten, we wake up by five or six, much more refreshed. This is important for all types as well as for Kapha. The nervous system heals itself during sleep, and digestion completes its processing during sleep as well.

- Weight Control: Kaphas may just look at food and gain weight, sad but true. This is why Kaphas need to adhere very closely to a diet that will reduce the Kapha Effect in their bodies. It helps to reduce sweets in the diet, as sweets increase Kapha and weight (see Chapters 10 and 11). Too much sweetness in the diet may also lead to diabetes, a Kapha disease.

Part IV: Exercises for Health and Well-Being

- Meditation: daily meditation can help to strengthen a Kapha's natural peaceful and contended nature. It is detoxification for the mind. Find the meditation technique most suitable to your lifestyle and disposition. It may be helpful to take a lesson or two.

- No Anger, No Worry: while Kapha is less prone to upset, anger, and anxiety, these emotions always create an imbalance in the body. Avoid situations that cause anger, worry and upset, which will aggravate any condition. If your job creates anger and upset, you may need to find a different job. If you are constantly worried about finances, you may need to reduce your overhead to reduce stress. If you are angry with someone, try to forgive.

- Avoid Late-Night Activities: when we begin a project in the early evening, we engage our mind and emotions for the intensity to follow through to the completion of whatever we are doing. This increases the Vata and Pitta Effect on our physiology, and will tend to keep us from falling asleep or having a peaceful night. The early evening should be the winding down part of the day as we decrease our more intense activities.

- Practicing Forgiveness: the physiology of forgiveness is more powerful than any other medicine. The physiology of resentment creates illness wherever it goes. Forgiveness is very healing; it reduces the Vata and Pitta Effect, which even Kaphas experience. According to Ayurveda, Kapha has the greater capacity for forgiveness, which may be due to their calmer, more peaceful nature.

- Sun Salutations: an exercise called Sun Salutations is an excellent way to start the day. These postures will add flexibility and strength to the body. Begin with up to six sets of Sun Salutations. Remember Kapha, *you need to exercise.*

- Rest During Menstrual Cycle (Female): Ayurveda teaches the importance of rest during the first day or so of a woman's menstrual cycle. If total rest is not practical, getting as much rest as possible during these days is a must. However, if you are working, your employer may not think it a good idea to stay home during this time, and you may not feel able to take days off and forfeit the income. However, do what you can; rest when you can.

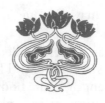

Chapter 15

SUMMARY

Concerns about our health have been with us forever, and will continue to be with us. The only path to a life well lived is to understand the rules of the game of life, or *natural law*. Natural law is the way the universe works. Our perceptions of these laws may vary from culture to culture, but the theme of wholism runs through all cultures. The ancient teachings of Ayurveda have the wholistic principle at their core. The concept of the Wholistic Principle, applied through Ayurveda, enables us to take an active role in improving and sustaining our health.

The natural laws regarding health are made much clearer when we understand the physiology of the body according to the three metabolic types. The three Ayurvedic body types (Vata, Pitta, Kapha) correlate with modern physiology to a high degree, providing insight beyond our current reductionist scientific approach. When we combine both the ancient wisdom of Ayurveda and the newest scientific protocols for diagnosis, the process of illness can be seen with much greater clarity.

Wholism and Ayurveda bring us other insights into the workings of the body: for instance, Vata body types (Metabolic Type I) require a different diet than Pitta (Type II) or Kapha (Type III) because the autonomic nervous system and hormone response to the ingestion of proteins, fats, and carbohydrates differ in each type. Through Ayurveda we may easily determine our genetic constitution (body type) and any imbalances we may suffer. When we then incorporate certain wholistic principles with ancient Ayurvedic practices, we are given the tools to balance our body/mind, gain control over our weight, and improve our overall health. By following a well-defined program of diet and daily practices for our particular body type, we can learn to nurture ourselves, thus achieving greater strength and insight for achieving our destiny.

BIBLIOGRAPHY

1.   Bohm, David; *Wholeness and the Implicate Order*; Ark
      Paperbacks, London and New York, 1980

2.   Capra, Fritjof; *The Tao of Physics*; Bantam Books, New
      York 1977

3.   Capra, Fritjof; *The Turning Point*; Bantam Books, New
      York 1988

4.   Chopra, Deepak, M.D.; *Perfect Health:* The Complete
      Mind/Body Guide; Harmony Books, New York 1991

5.   Chopra, Deepak, M.D.; *Unconditional Life*: Mastering the
      Forces That Shape Personal Reality; Bantam Books,
      New York 1991

6.   Erasmus, Udo; *Fats that Heal, Fats that Kill*; Alive Books,
      Burnaby, BC, Canada 1986,1993

7.   Erasmus, Udo; *Fats and Oils*: The Complete Guide to
      Fats and Oils in Health and Nutrition; Alive Books,
      Vancouver, Canada 1986

8.   Finckh, Elisabeth, M.D.; *Studies in Tibetan Medicine*;
      Snow Lion Publications, Ithaca, New York 1988

9.   Frawley, David; *Ayurvedic Healing*; Passage Press, Salt
      Lake City, Utah 1989

10.   Frawley, David; *The Astrology of Seers*; Passage Press, Salt
      Lake City, Utah 1990

11.   Garde, Dr. R.K.; *Ayurveda for Health and Long Life*; D.B.
      Taraporevala Sons & Co., Bombay, India 1975

12.   Gerson, Scott, M.D.; *Ayurveda: The Ancient Indian
      Healing Art*; Element Books Ltd., Shaftesbury, Dorset,
      England 1993

13. Guyton, Arthur C., M.D. and John E. Hall, Ph.D.; *Textbook of Medical Physiology*, Ninth Edition; W.B. Saunders Company, Philadelphia, Pennsylvania 1956-1996

14. Heyn, Birgit; *Ayurveda: The Ancient Indian Art of Natural Medicine & Life Extension*; Healing Arts Press, Rochester, Vermont 1990

15. Lad, Dr. Vasant; *Ayurveda: The Science of Self-Healing*; Lotus Press, Wisconsin 1984

16. Lad, Dr. Vasant, Dr. David Frawley; *The Yoga of Herbs*; Lotus Light Publishing, Wisconsin 1986

17. Langman, Jan, M.D., Ph.D.; *Medical Embryology*; Williams & Wilkins, Baltimore/London 1981

18. Luciano, Vander Sherman; *Human Physiology: The Mechanisms of Body Function*; McGraw-Hill, New York

19. McClintic, J. Robert, Ph.D.; *Basic Anatomy and Physiology of the Human Body*; John Wiley & Sons, Inc. 1975

20. Monte, Tom; *World Medicine: The East West Guide to Healing Your Body*; Jeremy P. Tarcher/Perigee Books 1993

21. Morningstar, Amadea; *Ayurvedic Cooking for Westerners*; Lotus Press, Twin Lakes, Wisconsin 1995

22. Ranade, Dr. Subhash; *Natural Healing Through Ayurveda*; Passage Press, Salt Lake City, Utah 1993

23. Schore, Allan N.; *Affect Regulation and the Origin of The Self*; Lawrence Erlbaum Associates, Hillsdale, New Jersey 1994

24. Sears, Barry, Ph.D.; *The Zone: A Dietary Road Map*; HarperCollins Books, New York 1995

25. Selye, Dr. Hans; *The Stress of Life*, McGraw-Hill, New York 1978

26. Sharma, Hari, M.D.; *Freedom from Disease*; Veda Publishing, Toronto, Ontario, Canada 1993

27. Sharma, Priyavrat, Editor-Translator; *Caraka-Samhita*; Chaukhambha Orientalia, Varanasi, India 1981

28. Snell, Richard S., M.D., Ph.D.; *Clinical Neuroanatomy for Medical Students*; Little, Brown & Company, Boston 1980

29. Svoboda, Dr. Robert E.; *Prakruti*; Geocom Ltd., Albuquerque, New Mexico 1989

30. Svoboda, Dr. Robert E; *Ayurveda: Life, Health and Longevity*; Penguin Books Ltd., Middlesex, England 1992

31. Tarabilda, Edward F.; *Ayurveda Revolutionized: Integrating Ancient and Modern Ayurveda*; Lotus Press, Twin Lakes, Wisconsin 1997

32. Tiwari, Maya; *A Life of Balance: The Complete Guide to Ayurvedic Nutrition and Body Types with Recipes*; Healing Arts Press, Rochester Vermont 1995

33. Verma, Dr. Vinod; *Ayurveda, A Way of Life;* Samuel Weiser, Inc., York Beach, Maine 1995

INFORMATION ABOUT
THE AUTHOR

The Colorado Holistic Center
Dr. Dennis Thompson, Chiropractic Physician

Holistic diagnosis including:
1. Integrated medical and chiropractic examination
2. Laboratory blood testing
3. Ayurvedic diagnosis
4. Body Type analysis

Services:
1. Chiropractic and Medical care
2. Women's Health Care
3. Supplemental Nutritional Therapy (herbs, enzymes, vitamins, Ayurvedic Remedies)
4. Ayurvedic Medicine
5. Life Style Management Program according to body type
6. Ayurvedic Rejuvenation and Detoxification Therapies (Pancha Karma)
7. Ayurvedic Spa Therapies

Dr. Dennis Thompson, along with a fully trained professional staff, works with you to provide a clear clinical diagnosis based on Ayurvedic and Western Medicine. The Colorado Holistic Center offers an extended week-long healing program of rejuvenation called Pancha Karma. They blend modern medicine and traditional holistic medicine to create a more advanced system of diagnosis and treatment which they call Exceptional Medicine.

To schedule a new patient interview to determine if you are a candidate for their exceptional health recovery program, call:

The Colorado Holistic Center

Dennis Thompson D.C.
Denver, CO
1-888-682-1600

Ayurvedic Zone Diet:

For information on seminars, services, consultations and products call:

Dr. Dennis Thompson
Chiropractic Physician
Ayurvedic Practitioner
1-800-601-9707
E-mail address: drtdrt@concentric.net

Resource List:

Ayurvedic Spa Medicine

Spa Medicine is wholistic health care delivered within a spa or retreat setting for the benefit of increased health recovery and healing.
Ayurvedic Spa Therapy and Facilities: Dr. Dennis Thompson and a fully trained professional staff work with you to provide clear clinical diagnosis based on Ayurvedic and Western medicine. They offer an extended healing program of rejuvenation called Pancha Karma, wholistic chiropractic care, as well as effective spa therapies specially designed to soothe and heal your MIND/BODY TYPE.

Ayurvedic Zone Diet seminars, consultations, and products available at 1-800-601-9707
E-mail address: drtdrt@concentric.net

Dr. Dennis Thompson
Chiropractic Physician
Ayurvedic Practitioner
1-800-601-9707

Aromatherapy Study Programs

Aromatherapy Video and Home Study Program
Michael Scholes
(founder of Aroma Vera)
3384 S. Robertson Place
Los Angeles, CA 90034
Ph: 800-677-2368

Jeanne Rose
Aromatherapy and
Herbal Healing
Intensives
Attn: Jeanne Rose
219 Carl Street
San Francisco, CA 94117

London School of
Aromatherapy
P.O. Box 780
London NW5 1DY
England

Pacific Institute of
Aromatherapy
Attn: Kurt Schnaubelt
P.O. Box 8723
San Rafael, CA 94903
Ph: 515-479-9121

Quintessence
Aromatherapy
Attn: Ann Berwick
P.O. Box 4996
Boulder, CO 80306
Ph: 303-258-3791

Ayurveda Centers and Programs

Australian Institute of
Ayurvedic Medicine
19 Bowey Avenue
Enfield S.A. 5085
Australia
Ph: 08-349-7303

Ayurveda for Radiant
Health & Beauty
16 Espira Court
Santa Fe, NM 87505
Ph: 505-466-7662

Ayurvedic Healing Arts
Center
16508 Pine Knoll Road
Grass Valley, CA 95945
Ph: 916-274-9000

Ayurvedic Holistic
Center
82A Bayville Ave.
Bayville, NY 11709

The Ayurvedic Institute
and Wellness Center
11311 Menaul, NE
Albuquerque, NM 87112
Ph: 505-291-9698
Fax: 505-294-7572

Ayurvedic Living
Workshops
P.O. Box 188
Exeter, Devon EX4 5AB
England

California College of
Ayurveda
1117A East Main street
Grass Valley, CA 95945
Ph: 530-274-9100
Web:
www.ayurvedacollege.com
E-Mail:
info@ayurvedacollege.com
Clinical training in
Ayurveda

Center for Mind, Body
Medicine
P.O. Box 1048
La Jolla, CA 92038
Ph: 619-794-2425

The Chopra Center for
Well Being
7590 Fay Avenue
Suite 403
LaJolla, CA 92037
Ph: 619-551-7788
Fax: 619-551-7811

John Douillard
Life Spa, Rejuvenation
through Ayur-Veda
3065 Center Green Dr.
Boulder CO 80301
Ph: 303-442-1164,
Fax: 303-442-1240

East West College of
Herbalism Ayurvedic
Program
Represents courses of
Dr. David Frawley and
Dr. Michael Tierra in
UK
Hartswood, Marsh
Green, Hartsfield
E. Sussex TN7 4ET
United Kingdom
Ph: 01342-822312
Fax: 01342-826346
E-Mail:
ewcolherb@aol.com

EverGreen Herb Garden
and Learning Center,
Candis Cantin Packard
PO Box 1445, Placerville
CA 95667
Ph. and Fax: 530-626-
9288
Email:
evrgreen@innercite.com

Himalayan Institute
RR1, Box 400
Honesdale, PA 18431
Ph: 800-822-4547

Inside Ayurveda
Bi-monthly, independent
publication for Ayurvedic
professionals.
Niika Quistgard
PO Box 3021, Quincy
CA 995971-3021
Ph: 530-283-3717
Email:
oflife@inreach.com

Institute for Wholistic
Education
33719 116th Street
Box AZD
Twin Lakes, WI 53181
Ph: 262-877-9396
Beginner and Advanced
Correspondence Courses
in Ayurveda

Integrated Health
Systems
3855 Via Nova Marie,
#302D
Carmel, CA 93923
Ph: 408-476-5130

International Academy
of Ayurved
NandNandan, Atreya
Rugnalaya
M.Y. Lele Chowk
Erandawana, Pune: 411
004 , India
Ph/Fax:
91-212-378532/524427
E-Mail:
avilele@hotmail.com

International Ayurvedic
Institute
111 Elm Street
Suite 103-105
Worcester, MA 01609
Ph: 508-755-3744
Fax: 508-770-0618
E-Mail:
ayurveda@hotmail.com

International Federation
of Ayurveda
Dr. Krishna Kumar
27 Blight Street
Ridleyton S.A. 5008
Australia
Ph: 08-346-0631

Life Impressions
Institute
Attn: Donald
VanHowten, Director
613 Kathryn Street
Santa Fe, NM 87501
Ph: 505-988-2627

Lotus Ayurvedic Center
4145 Clares Street
Suite D
Capitola, CA 95010
Ph: 408-479-1667

Maharishi Ayurved at the
Raj
1734 Jasmine Avenue
Fairfield, IA 52556
Ph: 800-248-9050
Fax: 515-472-2496

Maharishi Health Center
Hale Clinic
7 Park Crescent
London, W14 3H3
England

Natural Therapeutics
Center
'Surya Daya'
Gisingham, Nr. Iye
Suffolk, England

New England Institute
of Ayurvedic Medicine
111 N. Elm Street
Suites 103-105
Worcester, MA 01609
Ph: 508-755-3744
Fax: 508-770-0618
E-Mail:
ayurveda@hotmail.com

Rocky Mountain
Ayurvedic Health
Retreat
P.O. Box 5192
Pagosa Springs, CO
81147
Ph: 800-247-9654;
970-264-9224

Atreya Smith, Director
European Institute of
Vedic Studies
Ceven point N° 230
4 bis rue Taisson
30100 Ales, France
Fax (33) 466-60-53-72
Email:
Atreya@compuserve.com
www.atreya.com

Victoria Stern, N.D.
P.O. Box 1814
Laguna Beach, CA
92652
Ph: 714-494-8858

Vinayak Ayurveda
Center
2509 Virginia NE
Suite D
Albuquerque, NM 87110
Ph: 505-296-6522
Fax: 505-298-2932
Internet: www.ayur.com

Wise Earth School of
Ayurveda
Attn: Bri. Maya Tiwari
RR1 Box 484
Candler, NC 28715
Ph: 704-258-9999
Teachers and
Practitioners Training
Programs Only

Ayurvedic Cosmetic Companies

Auroma Int'l
P.O. Box 1008
Dept. AZD
Silver Lake, WI 53170
Ph: 262-889-8569
Fax: 262-889-8591
Importer and master distributor of Auroshikha
Incense, Chandrika
Ayurvedic Soap and
Herbal Vedic Ayurvedic
products

Bindi Facial Skin Care
A Division of Pratima Inc.
109-17 72nd Road
Lower Level
Forest Hills, New York
11375
Ph: 718-268-7348

Devi Inc. (for Shivani
product line)
Attn: Anjali Mahaldar
P.O. Box 377
Lancaster, MA 01523
Ph: 800-237-8221
Fax: 508-368-0455

Gajee Herbals
The Khenpo Company
Attn: Gayatri Puri,
Owner
17595 Harvard Street,
C531
Irvine, CA 92714
Ph: 714-250-6027

Internatural
33719 116th St.-AZD
Twin Lakes, WI 53181
USA
800-643-4221 (toll free
order line)
262-889-8581 (office
phone)
262-889-8591 (fax)
email:
internatural@lotuspress.com
web site:
www.internatural.com
Retail mail order and
internet reseller of essential oils, herbs, spices,
supplements, herbal
remedies, incense, books
and other supplies

Lotus Brands, Inc.
P.O. Box 325-AZD
Twin Lakes, WI 53181
Ph: 262-889-8561
Fax: 262-889-8591
email:
lotusbrands@lotuspress.com
Manufacturer and distributor of natural personal care and herbal
products, massage oils,
essential oils, incense and
aromatherapy items

Lotus Light Enterprises
P O Box 1008-AZD
Silver Lake, WI 53170
USA
800-548-3824 (toll free
order line)
262-889-8501 (office
phone)
262-889-8591 (fax)
email:
lotuslight@lotuspress.com
Wholesale distributor of
essential oils, herbs,
spices, supplements,
herbal remedies, incense,
books and other supplies.
must supply resale cer-
tificate number or practitioner license to obtain
catalog of more than
10,000 items.

Siddhi Ayurvedic Beauty
Products
C/O Vinayak Ayurveda
Center
2509 Virginia NE, Suite D
Albuquerque, NM 87110
Ph: 505-296-6522
Fax: 505-298-2932

Swami Sada Shiva Tirtha
Ayurvedic Holistic
Center
82A Bayville Avenue
Bayville, NY 11709
Ph/Fax: 516-628-8200

TEJ Beauty Enterprises,
Inc.
(an Ayurvedic Beauty
Salon)
162 West 56th Street
Room 201
New York, NY 10019
(owner: Pratima
Raichur, founder of
Bindi)
Ph: 212-581-8136

Ayurvedic Herbal Suppliers

Auroma Int'l
P.O. Box 1008
Dept. AZD
Silver Lake, WI 53170
Ph: 262-889-8569
fax: 262-889-8591
Importer and master dis-
tributor of Auroshikha
Incense, Chandrika
Ayurvedic Soap and
Herbal Vedic Ayurvedic
products

Ayur Herbal
Corporation
P.O. Box 6390 YA
Santa Fe, NM 87502
Ph: 262-889-8569

Ayush Herbs, Inc.
10025 N.E. 4th Street
Bellevue, WA 98004
Ph: 800-925-1371

Bazaar of India Imports,
Inc.
1810 University Avenue
Berkeley, CA 94703
Ph: 800-261-7662;
510-548-4110

Dhanvantri
Aushadhalaya
Herbs of Wisdom and
Love, Ayurvedic Herbs
and Classical Formulas.
PO Box 1654, San
Anselmo CA 94979
Ph: 415-289-7976
Email:
ayurveda@dhanvantri.com

Dr. Singha's Mustard
Bath and More
Attn: Anna Searles
Natural Therapeutic
Centre
2500 Side Cove
Austin, TX 78704
Ph: 800-856-2862

Bio Veda
215 North Route 303
Congers, NY 10920-
1726
Ph: 800-292-6002

Frontier Herbs
P.O. Box 229
Norway, IA 52318
Ph: 800-669-3275

HerbalVedic Products
P.O. Box 6390
Santa Fe, NM 87502

Internatural
33719 116th St.-AZD
Twin Lakes, WI 53181
USA
800-643-4221 (toll free
order line)
262-889-8581 (office
phone)
262-889-8591 (fax)
email:
internatural@lotuspress.com
web site:
www.internatural.com
Retail mail order and
internet reseller of essential oils, herbs, spices,
supplements, herbal
remedies, incense, books
and other supplies

Kanak
P.O. Box 13653
Albuquerque, NM
87192-3653
Ph: 505-275-2469

Lotus Brands, Inc.
P.O. Box 325-AZD
Twin Lakes, WI 53181
Ph: 262-889-8561
Fax: 262-889-8591
email:
lotusbrands@lotuspress.com
Manufacturer and distributor of natural personal care and herbal products, massage oils, essential oils, incense and aromatherapy items

Lotus Herbs
1505 42nd Avenue
Suite 19
Capitola, CA 95010
Ph: 408-479-1667

Lotus Light Enterprises
P O Box 1008-AZD
Silver Lake, WI 53170
USA
800-548-3824 (toll free order line)
262-889-8501 (office phone)
262-889-8591 (fax)
email:
lotuslight@lotuspress.com
Wholesale distributor of essential oils, herbs, spices, supplements, herbal remedies, incense, books and other supplies. must supply resale certificate number or practitioner license to obtain catalog of more than 10,000 items.

Maharishi Ayurveda
Products Intl., Inc.
417 Bolton Road
P.O. Box 541
Lancaster, MA 01523
Info: 800-843-8332
Order: 800-255-8332

Quantum Publication,
Inc.
P.O. Box 1088
Sudbury, MA 01776
Ph: 800-858-1808

Vinayak Panchakarma
Chikitsalaya
Y.M.C.A Complex,
Situbuldi
Nagpur (Maharastra
State)
India 440 012
Ph: 011-91-712-538983
Fax: 011-91-712-552409
Retail/Wholesale

Yoga of Life Center
2726 Tramway N.E.
Albuquerque, NM 87122
Ph: 505-275-6141

Bodywork Training

The Center For Release
and Integration
450 Hillside Drive
Mill Valley, CA 94941

Dr. Jay Scherer's
Academy of Natural
Healing
1443 St. Francis Drive
Santa Fe, NM 87505
The Rolf Institute
205 Canyon Blvd.
Boulder, CO 80302

The Upledger Institute
1211 Prosperity Farms
Road
Palm Beach Gardens, FL
33410

The Feldenkrais Guild
524 Ellsworth St. SW,
P.O. Box 489

Correspondence Courses

American Institute of
Vedic Studies
Dr. David Frawley,
Director
P.O. Box 8357
Santa Fe, NM
87504-8357
Ph: 505-983-9385
Fax: 505-982-5807
E-Mail:
vedicinst@aol.com
Web:
consciousnet.com/vedic
Correspondence courses
in Ayurveda and Vedic
Astrology

Lessons and Lectures in
Ayurveda by Dr. Robert
Svoboda
P.O. Box 23445
Albuquerque, NM
87192-1445
Ph: 505-291-9698

Institute for Wholistic
Education
33719 116th Street
Box AZD
Twin Lakes, WI 53181
Ph: 262-877-9396

To train in Ayurvedic Facial Massage and Beauty Practices

Melanie Sachs
"Invoking Beauty with
Ayurveda" Seminars
214 Girard Blvd., N.E.
Albuquerque, NM 87106
Ph: 505-265-4826

Beauty and Quality Ayurvedic Supplements

Auroma Int'l
P.O. Box 1008
Dept. AZD
Silver Lake, WI 53170
Ph: 262-889-8569
fax: 262-889-8591
Importer and master distributor of Auroshikha Incense, Chandrika Ayurvedic Soap and Herbal Vedic Ayurvedic products

Ayur Herbal Corporation
P.O. Box 6390 YA
Santa Fe, NM 87502
Ph: 262-889-8569
fax: 262-889-8591
Manufacturer of Herbal Vedic Ayurvedic products

Internatural
33719 116th St.-AZD
Twin Lakes, WI 53181
USA
800-643-4221 (toll free order line)
262-889-8581 (office phone)
262-889-8591 (fax)
email:
internatural@lotuspress.com
web site:
www.internatural.com
Retail mail order and internet reseller of essential oils, herbs, spices, supplements, herbal remedies, incense, books and other supplies

Lotus Brands, Inc
P.O. Box 325-AZD
Twin Lakes, WI 53181
Ph: 262-889-8561
Fax: 262-889-8591
email:
lotusbrands@lotuspress.com
Manufacturer and distributor of natural personal care and herbal products, massage oils, essential oils, incense and aromatherapy items

Lotus Light Enterprises
P O Box 1008-AZD
Silver Lake, WI 53170
USA
800-548-3824 (toll free order line)
262-889-8501 (office phone)
262-889-8591 (fax)
email:
lotuslight@lotuspress.com
Wholesale distributor of essential oils, herbs, spices, supplements, herbal remedies, incense, books and other supplies. must supply resale certificate number or practitioner license to obtain catalog of more than 10,000 items.

Maharishi Ayur-Veda Products International, Inc.
417 Bolton Road
P.O. Box 54
Lancaster, MA 01523
Ph: 800-ALL-VEDA
Fax: 508-368-7475

New Moon Extracts
P.O. Box 1947
Brattleborough, Vermont 05302-1947
Ph: 800-543-7279

Spectrum Natural
Omega 3 Oil
The Oil Company
133 Copeland Street
Petaluma, CA 94952

Color, Sound, and Gems

PAZ
P.O. Box 4859
Albuquerque, NM 87196
For open-backed gemstone settings

Color Therapy Eyewear
C/O Terri Perrigone-Messer
P.O. Box 3114
Diamond Springs, CA 95619

Lumatron (light device)
C/O Ernie Baker
515 Pierce Street #3
San Francisco, CA 94117
Ph: 415-626-0083

Genesis (sound device)
Medical Massage Therapy
Attn: Tina Shinn
1857 Northwest Blvd.
Annex
Columbus, Ohio 43212
Ph: 614-488-5244

Essential Oil Supplies

Aromatherapy Supply
Unit W3
The Knoll Business
Center
Old Shoreham Road
Hove, Sussex BN3 7GS
England

Aroma Vera
3384 S. Robertson Place
Los Angeles, CA 90034
Ph: 800-669-9514

Auroma Int'l
P.O. Box 1008
Dept. AZD
Silver Lake, WI 53170
Ph: 262-889-8569
fax: 262-889-8591
importer and master distributor of Auroshikha Incense, Chandrika Ayurvedic Soap and Herbal Vedic Ayurvedic products

Fenmail Tisserand Oils
P.O. Box 48
Spalding, LINCS PE11
ADS
England

Internatural
33719 116th St.-AZD
Twin Lakes, WI 53181
USA
800-643-4221 (toll free order line)
262-889-8581 (office phone)
262-889-8591 (fax)
email:
internatural@lotuspress.com
web site:
www.internatural.com
Retail mail order and
internet reseller of essential oils, herbs, spices, supplements, herbal remedies, incense, books and other supplies

Lotus Brands, Inc.
P.O. Box 325-AZD
Twin Lakes, WI 53181
Ph: 262-889-8561
Fax: 262-889-8591
email:
lotusbrands@lotuspress.com
Manufacturer and distributor of natural personal care and herbal products, massage oils, essential oils, incense and aromatherapy items

Lotus Light Enterprises
P O Box 1008-AZD
Silver Lake, WI 53170
USA
800-548-3824 (toll free order line)
262-889-8501 (office phone)
262-889-8591 (fax)
email:
lotuslight@lotuspress.com
Wholesale distributor of essential oils, herbs, spices, supplements, herbal remedies, incense, books and other supplies. must supply resale certificate number or practitioner license to obtain catalog of more than 10,000 items.

Private Universe
P.O. Box 3122
Winter Park, FL 32790
Ph: 407-644-7203

Oshadi Ayus - Quality
Life Products
15, Monarch Bay Plaza
Suite 346
Monarch Beach, CA
92629
Ph: 800-947-1008
Fax: 714-240-1104

Primavera
D 8961 Sulzberg
Germany
08376-808-0

Original Swiss Aromatics
P.O. Box 606
San Rafael, CA 94915
Ph: 415-459-3998

Exercise Programs and Information

Callanetic Headquarters
1700 Broadway
Suite 2000
Denver, CO 80290
Ph: 303-831-4455

Diamond Way Health
Associates
214 Girard Blvd. NE
Albuquerque, NM 87106
Ph: 505-265-4826
(for Sotai, Tibetan Rejuvenation Exercises)

Vega Study Center
1511 Robinson Street
Oroville, CA 95965
Ph: 916-533-7702
(for Sotai instructions - books)

Satori Resources
732 Hamlin Way
San Leandro, CA 94578
(for Tai Chi Chih)

Kushi Institute
P.O. Box 7
Becket, MA 01223
Ph: 413-623-5741
(for Do-in)

Natural Ingredients

Aloe Farms
Box 125
Los Fresnos, TX 78566
Ph: 800-262-6771
(for aloe vera juice, gel,
powder and capsules)

Arya Laya Skin Care
Center
Rolling Hills Estates, CA
90274
(for carrot oil)

Aubrey Organics
4419 North Manhattan
Avenue
Tampa, FL 33614
(for rosa mosquita oil
and a large variety of
natural cosmetics and
shampoos)

Body Shop
45 Horsehill Road
Cedar Knolls, NJ
07927-2014
Ph: 800-541-2535
(aloe vera, nut and seed
oils, cosmetics, make-up,
brushes, loofahs, and
much more)

Culpepper Ltd.
21 Bruton Street
London W1X 7DA
England
(variety of natural seed,
nut, and kernal oils,
essential oils, herbs,
books, and cosmetics)

Desert Whale Jojoba Co.
P.O. Box 41594
Tucson, AZ 85717
Ph: 602-882-4195
(for jojoba products and
many other natural oils,
including rice bran,
pecan, macadamia nut
and apricot kernal)

Everybody Ltd.
1738 Pearl Street
Boulder, CO 80302
Ph: 800-748-5675
(large variety of oils, oil
blends, and cosmetics)

Flora Inc.
P.O. Box 950
805 East Badger Road
Lynden, WA 98264
Ph: 800-446-2110
(for flax seed oil, herbal
supplements for skin,
hair, nails and cosmetics)

Green Earth Farm
P.O. Box 672
65 1/2 North 8th Street
Saguache, CO 81149
(for calendula oil, creme,
and herbal bath)

The Heritage Store, Inc.
P.O. Box 444
Virginia Beach, VA
23458
Ph: 804-428-0100
(castor oil, organic ghee,
cocoa butter, massage
oils, flowerwaters, essential oils, cosmetics, and
natural home remedies)

Internatural
33719 116th St.-AZD
Twin Lakes, WI 53181
USA
800-643-4221 (toll free
order line)
262-889-8581 (office
phone)
262-889-8591 (fax)
email:
internatural@lotuspress.com
web site:
www.internatural.com
Retail mail order and
internet reseller of essential oils, herbs, spices,
supplements, herbal
remedies, incense, books
and other supplies

Janca's Jojoba Oil and
Seed Company
456 E. Juanita #7
Mesa, AZ 85204
Ph: 602-497-9494
(jojoba oil, butter, wax,
and seeds. Also a large
variety of naturally
pressed unusual oils,
such as camellia, kukui
nut, and grapeseed. Also
have clay, aloe products,
essential oils, and their
own line of cosmetics)

Lotus Brands, Inc.
P.O. Box 325-AZD
Twin Lakes, WI 53181
Ph: 262-889-8561
Fax: 262-889-8591
email:
lotusbrands@lotuspress.com
Manufacturer and dis-
tributor of natural per-
sonal care and herbal
products, massage oils,
essential oils, incense and
aromatherapy items

Lotus Light Enterprises
P O Box 1008-AZD
Silver Lake, WI 53170
USA
800-548-3824 (toll free
order line)
262-889-8501 (office ph.)
262-889-8591 (fax)
email:
lotuslight@lotuspress.com
Wholesale distributor of
essential oils, herbs,
spices, supplements,
herbal remedies, incense,
books and other supplies.
must supply resale cer-
tificate number or practitioner license to obtain
catalog of more than
10,000 items.

Weleda, Inc.
841 South Main Street
Spring Valley, NY 10977
(for calendula oil and a
large variety of natural
cosmetics)

Non-Denominational Meditation Training

Shambhala Training
International
Executive Offices
1084 Tower Road
Halifax, Nova Scotia
Canada B3H 265

Organic Milk/Certified Raw Milk Suppliers

Alta Delta Certified Raw
Milk
P.O. Box 388
City of Industry, CA
91747
Ph: 818-964-6401
(non pasteurized, non-
homogenized milk)

Natural Horizons, Inc.
7490 Clubhouse Road
Boulder, CO 80301
Ph: 303-530-2711
(organic/pasteurized,
non-homogenized milk;
whole, low-fat, skim but-
termilk and cream)

Organic Valley Family of
Farms
C/O Cropp Cooperative
La Farge, WI
Ph: 608-625-2602
(organic butter, non-
homogenized low-fat milk)

Pancha Karma Kitchen Equipment

Earth Fare
Attn: Roger Derrough
66 Westgate parkway
Asheville, NC 28806
Ph: 704-253-7656
Carries hand grinders
and suribachi clay pots
and bowls.

Garber Hardware
49 Eighth Avenue
New York, NY 10014
Carries hand grinders,
but no mail order.

Sesam Muhle Natural
Products
RR1
Durham, Ontario
Canada, NOG 1RO
Ph: 519-369-6326
Carries a line of hand
grinders and flakers for
grains and legumes,
made in Germany.

Taj Mahal Imports
1594 Woodcliff Drive,
N.E.
Atlanta, GA 30329
Ph: 404-321-5940
Carries a full line of
Indian kitchen equip-
ment.

Pancha Karma Supplies

Vicki Stern
P.O. Box 1814
Laguna Beach, CA
92651
Ph: 714-494-8858
(for steam boxes)

To Receive Pancha Karma

The Colorado Holistic
Center
Dennis Thompson D.C.
Denver, CO
1-888-682-1600

Diamond Way Health
Associates
214 Girard Blvd., NE
Albuquerque, NM 87106
Ph: 505-265-4826

Dr. Lobsang Rapgay
2931 Tilden Ave.
Los Angeles, CA 90064
Ph: 310-477-3877

Ayurvedic Spa Medicine

Ancient Way Ayurvedic
Health Spa
Attn: Dr. Dennis
Thompson
800-601-9707
E-Mail:
drtdrt@concentric.net

Vedic Astrology

American Council of
Vedic Astrology (ACVA)
PO Box 2149
Sedona, AZ 86339
Ph: 800-900-6595;
520-282-6595
Fax: 520-282-6097
Web:
www.vedicastrology.org
E-Mail:
acva@sedona.net
Conferences, tutorial and
training programs

American Institute of
Vedic Studies
Dr. David Frawley,
Director
P.O. Box 8357
Santa Fe, NM 87504-
8357
Ph: 505-983-9385
Fax: 505-982-5807
E-Mail:
vedicinst@aol.com
Web:
consciousnet.com/vedic
Correspondence courses
in Ayurveda and Vedic
Astrology

Videos

Feldenkrais Resources
Ph: 800-765-1907

Wishing Well Video
P.O. Box 1008
Dept. AZD
Silver Lake, WI 53170
Ph: 262-889-8501
(wholesale & retail)

Index